Praise for *Supporting People to Live Well with Dementia*

'Sarah's book gives much-needed insight into how library services can provide well-designed and appropriately compassionate access to the library for people living with dementia and their carers. In considering the wide variety of creative resources and practices available when working with people with dementia, Sarah shows how libraries can become truly inclusive spaces.

The book provides an accessible account of the impacts of dementia on everyday life and considers how library services might respond to these impacts. By focusing on putting the person with dementia at the centre, the book highlights simple and meaningful principles that can be practically implemented.'
Dr Liz Brewster, Senior Lecturer, Lancaster Medical School

'This is a clear, well-written book highlighting the many benefits libraries can bring to people living with dementia and their carers. By using case studies and writing about the diverse methods adopted, Sarah demonstrates how libraries can support these customers. She emphasises the value of involving people with dementia and their carers, and of using techniques to fit the person.

The book shows the author's knowledge of dementia and the importance of gaining the views of people from this group, whenever possible. We will definitely be recommending this book.'
Betty Machin, Manager, Dementia advocacy project, Beth Johnson Foundation

Supporting People to Live Well with Dementia

Every purchase of a Facet book helps to fund CILIP's advocacy, awareness and accreditation programmes for information professionals.

Supporting People to Live Well with Dementia

A Guide for Library Services

Sarah McNicol

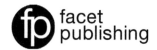

© Sarah McNicol 2023

Published by Facet Publishing
c/o British Library, 96 Euston Road, London NW1 2DB
www.facetpublishing.co.uk

Facet Publishing is wholly owned by CILIP:
the Library and Information Association.

The author has asserted her right under the Copyright, Designs and Patents Act 1988 to be identified as author of this work.

Except as otherwise permitted under the Copyright, Designs and Patents Act 1988 this publication may only be reproduced, stored or transmitted in any form or by any means, with the prior permission of the publisher, or, in the case of reprographic reproduction, in accordance with the terms of a licence issued by The Copyright Licensing Agency. Enquiries concerning reproduction outside those terms should be sent to Facet Publishing,
c/o British Library, 96 Euston Road, London NW1 2DB.

Every effort has been made to contact the holders of copyright material reproduced in this text, and thanks are due to them for permission to reproduce the material indicated. If there are any queries, please contact the publisher.

British Library Cataloguing in Publication Data
A catalogue record for this book is available from the British Library.

ISBN 978-1-78330-597-1 (paperback)
ISBN 978-1-78330-598-8 (hardback)
ISBN 978-1-78330-599-5 (PDF)
ISBN 978-1-78330-600-8 (EPUB)

First published 2023

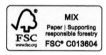

Typeset from author's files by Flagholme Publishing Services in
10/13 pt Palatino Linotype and Open Sans.
Printed and made in Great Britain by CPI Group (UK) Ltd, Croydon, CR0 4YY.

For the staff at Belong Crewe, particularly everyone on Britannia Household, who cared for my dad, James.

Contents

About the Author	xi
Preface	xiii
Acknowledgements	xvii
Introduction	**xix**
History and prevalence of dementia	xix
Public attitudes towards dementia	xxi
What does this mean for libraries?	xxiv
Supporting people to live well with dementia	xxvi
Scope and terminology	xxvii
1 What is Dementia?	**1**
Types of dementia	2
Stages of dementia	9
Understanding dementia	10
Potential impacts on the use of library services	14
Person-centred care	15
Conclusions	19
2 Supporting People Living with Dementia and their Carers	**21**
Social model of disability	22
Supporting library customers with dementia and their carers	28
Support for library staff affected by dementia	33
Training opportunities	36
Conclusions	39
3 Library Design and Environment	**41**
Finding the library	43
Getting around the library	43
Case studies of dementia-friendly library design	47
Sensory spaces	53
Conclusion: maintaining dementia-friendly library design	54

4	**Reading and Dementia**	**57**
	Dementia and imagination	58
	Dementia-friendly reading materials	60
	Reading activities for people with dementia and carers	69
	Conclusions	78
5	**Health, Social and Arts Activities**	**81**
	Health and therapy-informed activities	81
	Activities supporting social connections	86
	Arts-related activities	92
	Conclusions	99
6	**Digital and Online Provision**	**101**
	Online activity provision for people with dementia	102
	Other technologies for people with dementia	105
	Online provision for carers	107
	Conclusions	109
7	**Partnership Working**	**111**
	General partnership schemes	112
	Library-specific partnership schemes	113
	Conclusions	120
8	**Communications and Marketing**	**121**
	Language and terminology	122
	Design of communications materials	125
	Working with the media and other partners	127
	Conclusions	127
9	**Evaluation and Service Development**	**129**
	Key concepts	130
	Recruiting participants	130
	Evaluation and research methods	132
	Ethics	140
	Conclusions	141
10	**Future Trends**	**143**
	Demographic changes	143
	Conclusion: future library provision for people with dementia and their carers	152

Summary: ten actions for dementia-friendly libraries	**155**
References	**157**
Annotated Bibliography	**171**
Index	**179**

About the Author

Sarah McNicol has been a researcher since 2000, working on over 70 research and evaluation projects of differing scales and across a number of disciplines. She has worked for Manchester Metropolitan University (education), Birmingham City University (information studies), University of Leicester (health sciences) and Loughborough University (information studies), as well as on a freelance basis. She has also worked as a school librarian and as a tutor within the further and adult education sectors.

Sarah has a range of research interests and has published widely within the information sector and beyond, including two edited collections published by Facet Publishing: *Bibliotherapy* (2018) and *Critical Literacy for Information Professionals* (2016). In recent years, her research has focused on arts for health, bibliotherapy and community engagement in libraries and other cultural organisations. In particular, she has carried out research exploring how arts, culture and community organisations can support people with dementia and their carers. This has included co-creating a comic with a group of people with dementia; evaluating a shared reading programme for carers; and research into a bibliotherapy project operating in care homes.

Preface

My dad's experience of dementia wasn't the 'gradual decline' that's often used to describe the condition. With hindsight, he had started to have minor problems over a few months, but was living independently at home, and with no concerns about dementia, until he had a bad fall and ended up in hospital. He was there for four months, moved around between seven wards and three hospitals. I first realised he might have dementia when I visited him shortly after he was admitted. He thought he was at the steelworks where he had worked over 40 years earlier and wanted me to go into the office and get some paperwork he needed.

During the time he was in hospital, doctors would refer to dad's dementia, but no steps were taken to make a formal diagnosis – that only happened after he moved to a care home. Although I visited every other day, communication from the hospital was poor and the long stay certainly didn't improve his condition – physically or mentally. Support for me as his only close relative was non-existent. Early in his stay, there was an expectation that he would return home, possibly with adaptations to his house to accommodate his needs. But as time went on, it became clear this wasn't going to work.

Luckily, I had been doing research around dementia for a few years before this, in particular working with the Beth Johnson Foundation in Stoke-on-Trent and their peer support group for people with early- to mid-stage dementia, facilitated by dementia advocates. I'd learnt a lot from this group and had a much better idea than I might otherwise have done about what I was (and wasn't!) looking for in a care home for my dad. Homes I looked at were certainly varied, but I was lucky in finding one close to home which seemed welcoming and where staff had a positive approach to dementia and to care more broadly.

My dad lived at Belong Village in Crewe for two years until he died in June 2020. During those years, we had some of the best times together we'd had for many years. After he was made redundant from the steelworks in the late 1970s, dad had a hardware shop where he worked until he was 79. He was used to being around people and chatting with his customers. Retirement had been difficult – he'd put it off for as long as possible. Moving into a care home gave him back much of that companionship and gave him new people to get to know and build genuine relationships with. It also gave me people with whom I could share the experience of caring for dad. As Tom Kitwood, the researcher who pioneered much of our current understandings of dementia care, emphasised, human beings need others to share the task of caring – practically and emotionally; we are not 'designed' to do this alone (Kitwood, 1997, 41).

Unlike many descriptions of people with dementia 'losing themselves', my dad certainly didn't lose his personality; he could still be thoughtful, charming and funny – just as he could still be grumpy, stubborn and a terminal procrastinator at times. The difference was that he often gave free reign to aspects of his personality he'd previously kept more in check. Many of the other residents in dad's 'household' had more advanced dementia than him, but they also still had very definite and strong personalities; each had their own concerns, interests and preferences. Whether they were recognisable to people who had known them throughout their lives as the individuals they'd been previously, I don't know; but they were certainly not 'zombies' (Behuniak, 2011).

As someone who had always been quite set in his ways, dad became more open to new experiences (sometimes!). We did things I never thought he would have been open to, such as a music session (described in Chapter 5) and a movement workshop – neither of which I could have imagined him enjoying a few years before. I became aware that losses or gaps in his memory seemed to be compensated for by greater reliance on his imagination. Where memory ends and imagination begins can often be blurred for all of us, but dementia makes this blurring more palpable and perhaps lets us reach imaginative spaces we might not have done if we were constantly being drawn back to focus on conventional 'truths'.

This book is therefore based on the idea that living well with dementia is possible – with the right support. As organisations central to the life of many communities, libraries have a potentially vital role to play in supporting people with dementia and their carers. I continue to mention my dad at various points during this book. I have done this deliberately as a reminder that 'people with dementia' are not a homogenous group without feelings or opinions, but unique human beings with their own preferences, needs and foibles.

The COVID-19 pandemic has been a challenging time for people with dementia – in care homes and in the community. A review of published research concerning the impact of COVID-19 on the care and quality of life of people living with dementia and their carers found that the outbreak and subsequent enforced prolonged conditions of social isolation affected behavioural and psychological symptoms and Quality of Life (QoL) amongst people with dementia (Masterson-Algar et al., 2021). More specifically, studies have reported on negative impacts on memory, orientation abilities and concentration, as well as increased apathy, anxiety, agitation, aggression and depression amongst people with dementia (Alzheimer's Society, 2020; Canevelli et al., 2020; El Haj et al., 2020; Manca et al., 2020; Simonetti et al., 2020; Suárez-González et al., 2020). Carers were also affected, finding themselves more isolated and exposed to increased levels of stress (Alzheimer's Society, 2020; Canevelli et al. 2020; Cohen et al., 2020; Savla et al., 2021; Vaitheswaran et al., 2020).

This book was written during the second half of 2021 and the first half of 2022. During this period, many services offered by libraries before the pandemic were still not running or were only partially running. Some examples described in the book are therefore based on the pre-Covid situation, with the hope that these can continue to be offered in a similar format at a later date. However, the pandemic has also highlighted future possibilities for library services, such as the expansion of online provision introduced when public buildings were forced to close or limit access. I therefore also explore examples of online services introduced since 2020 to provide suggestions on when and how these can work successfully for people with dementia. Whilst, in some ways, writing a book about libraries and dementia at this time was not ideal, COVID-19 has made the need for community support – through libraries alongside other organisations – for people with dementia and their carers more urgent than ever. I hope that this book provides ideas, encouragement and inspiration to any library staff wishing to make their buildings, services and interactions with customers more inclusive of people with dementia and their carers.

Acknowledgements

With many thanks to everyone who supported me in writing this book:

Abby Wolfe, Public Awareness Co-ordinator, Alzheimer Society of Saskatchewan, Canada
Ann-Louise Vonk, Branch Librarian – Hāwera, South Taranaki District Council, New Zealand
Caroline Varney-Bowers, Community Librarian, Norfolk Library and Information Service, UK
Charlotte Sumner, Paignton Library, Libraries Unlimited, UK
Colin Robson, Community Cultural Development Coordinator, Durham County Council, UK
Elaine Duffy, former Co-ordinator, Words in Mind, UK
Elisabeth Marrow, Marlborough District Libraries, New Zealand
Ellen Wasserfall, Centre for Professional Development and Research, Health Agency, City of Oslo, Norway
Gwyneth Davies, Volunteers Co-ordinator, The National Library of Wales
Heather Cowie, National Project Manager, Dementia-Friendly Canada
Heather Rodenhurst, Team Librarian, Shropshire Council Library Service, UK
Jackie Burgess, Community and Outreach Librarian, Guille-Allès Library, Guernsey
Jackie Manners, Principal Librarian Wellbeing, Library Service, West Sussex County Council, UK
Julie Scanlon, retired university lecturer
Karen Morris, Health and Well Being Librarian, Stockton-on-Tees Borough Council, UK
Koren Calder, Reading Communities Outreach Manager, Scottish Book Trust

Laura Yates, Head of Participation, Bluecoat, Liverpool, UK
Lesley Davies, Sefton Libraries, UK
Liz Askew, Walsall Healthcare NHS Trust, UK
Lynsey Ilett, Customer Services Development Librarian, Folkestone & Hythe District, Libraries, Registration & Archives, Kent County Council, UK
Mari Gudim Torp, Deichman Oppsal Library, Norway
Mark Rathbone, Project Advisor, LiveWire, UK
Matthew Entwistle, Community Librarian, LiveWire, UK
Melody Schuetz, Head of Adult Services, North Shore Library, Glendale, US
Pamela Tulloch, Scottish Library and Information Council
Sara Griffiths, The National Archives, UK
Stephen Royle, Belper Library, UK
Stroma Mauritzen, National Librarian, Dementia Australia
Tabitha Moses, Project Facilitator, Where the Arts Belong, Bluecoat, Liverpool, UK
Trudy Jones, Library Development Officer, Halton Borough Council, UK

Introduction

Dementia is a condition that can have a profound impact on an individual and on their family and friends. Traditionally, the focus for dementia care has been medical treatments and care services. Increasingly, however, there is a focus on how we can enable people who have been diagnosed with dementia to live as full a life as possible, and encourage communities to work together to help people to stay healthier for longer. This means that libraries, alongside other services and organisations, have a potentially critical role to play in supporting people with dementia and their carers. This book aims to help library staff across a variety of sectors to gain a better understanding of the different ways in which library customers may be affected by dementia, and how people with dementia can continue to contribute positively to their communities. It presents ideas for ways in which libraries can better support people with dementia and their carers through approaches to customer service, design, resources, reading interventions and a range of other activities, as well as prompting more positive and inclusive attitudes towards people living with dementia amongst library staff, customers and communities more widely.

History and prevalence of dementia

Although there is evidence of an awareness of dementia since ancient times, the first modern recorded use of the word 'dementia' as a medical term is thought to be by Dr Philippe Pinel in 1797 (Torack, 1983). In 1906, German physician Alois Alzheimer made a significant breakthrough in understanding dementia. He inspected the brain of a deceased woman whom he had known to experience aggression, paranoia and memory problems that began when she was 50. Alzheimer discovered there was damage to the cerebral cortex of her brain from what he called 'tangles' and 'plaques'. This type of dementia was named Alzheimer's disease in 1909 (Ryan et al., 2015). Around the same time, German-born American neurologist Frederic Lewy discovered abnormal protein deposits in the brains of people with Parkinson's disease and identified what would become known as Lewy body dementia (Rodrigues e Silva et al., 2010).

However, despite these important breakthroughs, for the first three-quarters of the 20th century, there was relatively little interest in dementia in scientific circles. The person who probably did most to change perceptions was neurologist Robert Katzman. Katzman's 1976 landmark editorial 'The Prevalence and Malignancy of Alzheimer's Disease', published in *Archives of Neurology*, attracted the attention of medical and scientific communities. In a relatively short space of time, Alzheimer's disease went from being viewed as a relatively rare condition to a major public health issue. Today, the World Health Organization (WHO) recognises dementia as a global public health priority; it developed a Global Action Plan in 2017 and has established a Global Dementia Observatory (WHO, 2021).

Worldwide, there were an estimated 55 million people living with dementia in 2021 and there are 10 million new cases each year (WHO, 2021). To put the numbers into perspective, 10 million people is roughly the entire population of a country such as Sweden. It is difficult to calculate precise figures because the majority of the people with dementia globally have no formal diagnosis and, as a consequence, have limited access to information, support, care and treatment.

In the UK alone, an estimated 900,000 people are living with dementia (Alzheimer's Society, 2021), including over 42,000 below the age of 65 (ARUK, 2022). There are over 200,000 new cases of dementia in the UK each year (SCIE, 2020a). Around one in every 79 of the entire UK population, and one in 14 of the population aged 65 and over, has dementia and more than half the UK public knows someone who has been diagnosed with dementia (ARUK, 2022). Worryingly, only 58% of people with dementia in the UK say they are living well (Alzheimer's Society, 2014). Around 40% of people with dementia in the UK live in a care home, with around 80% of people in care homes having dementia or severe memory problems (SCIE, 2020a). This means 60% of people with dementia live in their own homes and, consequently, unpaid family carers provide a major part of the support. There are over 700,000 unpaid carers of people with dementia in the UK (SCIE, 2020a). Women are disproportionately affected by dementia, both in terms of developing the condition and in acting as unpaid carers (ARUK, 2015).

Statistics available elsewhere demonstrate that the issues are similar worldwide. In the United States, for instance, an estimated 6.2 million Americans aged 65 and older were living with Alzheimer's disease in 2021. By 2050, this number could rise to as high as 13 million (Alzheimer's Association, 2021). In Australia, there are estimated to be between 386,200 and 472,000 people living with dementia and the number is expected to reach over 849,300 by 2058. One in 12 Australians over 65 has dementia, and two in five of those over 90. It is estimated that between 134,900 and 337,200 people in Australia provide unpaid care for someone with dementia (AIHW, 2021).

Public attitudes towards dementia

In the late 20th and early 21st centuries, there has been an increase in the visibility of dementia in the public arena, both in terms of high-profile events, such as the G8 Summit on Dementia in 2013 and also in the media, and through sustained public awareness campaigns at national and local levels. Nevertheless, a lack of awareness and understanding of dementia remains a major concern around the world. Despite the rising profile of dementia, stigma associated with the condition continues to be a substantial problem. Stigma devalues a person as the individual is 'reduced in our minds from a whole and usual person to a tainted, discounted one' (Goffman, 1963, 3). It is commonplace to hear people with dementia and their families and carers say that a diagnosis has resulted in stigma and increasing social isolation. Perhaps this should not be altogether surprising as it is only over the last few decades that there has been a greater understanding of dementia as a chronic disease and a move by some dementia organisations to actively promote inclusivity.

Although some commentators argue that there has been a change in attitudes towards dementia during the first two decades of the 21st century, public fear of the condition is still widely reported. For example, surveys suggest that people over the age of 55 fear being diagnosed with dementia more than any other condition (Alzheimer's Society, 2016). In Alzheimer's Disease International's (ADI) 2012 survey on overcoming stigma, 75% of respondents thought that there was a stigma around people with Alzheimer's disease (Batsch and Mittelman, 2012). Stigma can take many different forms, including affording a low priority to an individual's quality of life, exclusion from social activities or avoiding a diagnosis (Bamford et al., 2014). People with dementia often lose their social networks and run the risk of isolation. They may also have difficulty in accessing support services, suffer from poor self-image and experience discrimination. Around one in four people with dementia hide or conceal their diagnosis, citing stigma as the main reason, and 40% of people with dementia report not being included in everyday life (Batsch and Mittelman, 2012).

Data from a survey by Dementia Australia show that 63% of people living with dementia and 73% of family, friends or carers surveyed believe discrimination against people living with dementia is common or very common. This includes families and friends dropping off and people with dementia reporting they are less likely to be included in social occasions and engagement. In addition, 55% of professionals surveyed believe that a doctor will often or always speak to the carer or support person rather than the person with dementia themselves, making an assumption that the person with the diagnosis no longer has the capacity to contribute to a conversation and/or make decisions for themselves. Of those living with dementia, 87% felt that people patronise them and treat them as if they are not smart (Dementia Australia, 2021a).

In addition to reports from people with dementia and carers, there is evidence of stigma towards people with dementia in research involving members of the general public. In a Canadian market research survey, 51% of those surveyed admitted to using some type of stigmatising language, such as telling dementia-related jokes. Half of all respondents did not believe that they could live well with dementia and more than one-quarter (27%) believed that their life would be over if they had dementia. 67% said they would feel uncomfortable disclosing their dementia to co-workers, and 55% and 46% respectively would feel uncomfortable disclosing to friends and to family members. This is perhaps unsurprising given that the same survey found that only 39% would offer support for family or friends who were open about their diagnosis and 36% would be uncomfortable interacting with a stranger who has dementia. This survey also highlighted the ways in which carers of people with dementia can struggle. One in five caregivers surveyed agreed that they sometimes feel embarrassed to be seen in public with the person they care for. 41% of caregivers believed that their life would be better if they were not caring for someone living with dementia, and two-thirds found the experience of caring for someone with dementia to be isolating (Alzheimer Society of Canada, 2017).

Cultural representations of dementia

As the level of stigma described above suggests, empathising with people with dementia is often not easy for those of us who do not have the condition. Gaining factual knowledge about the symptoms of dementia is helpful but can only go so far; understanding the experiences of people living with dementia, and using this knowledge to support then effectively, also requires imagination.

In recent years, there has been increasing interest in cultural representations of dementia, contributing to greater public awareness of the condition across the mainstream press, television, film, literature and other forms of art and media. However, cultural representations of people with dementia still often have a very negative focus and outlook. Whilst the experience of dementia can of course be a difficult one for both the person with dementia and their carers, when my dad was diagnosed with dementia, for the most part, I found the types of narratives widely available did not reflect my experiences or – as far as I could tell – his experiences either.

A review of research into depictions of dementia in popular culture across several countries found that the prevalent depictions involved negative images and feelings, and social distance between people with dementia and those without. Often, the person with dementia is depicted as without a voice and even not fully human. According to this study, the predominant emotion associated with dementia is fear (Low and Purwaningrum, 2020).

In addition, in many cultural representations, more attention is paid to the experiences of carers than to the experiences of those with dementia themselves – perhaps precisely because it is so difficult for people who do not have dementia to understand what living with the condition would be like. As dementia practice and research have progressed, the need to actively involve people with dementia has increasingly been recognised. However, it is still the case that people living with dementia are rarely given the opportunity of speaking for themselves; more usually, someone such as a family member or carer speaks on their behalf. As a result, discussions about, and portrayals of, dementia often emphasise the 'burden' that the illness can exert on the family, rather than the experiences of the person with dementia. In addition, it is worth noting that the majority of portrayals of dementia in the media and arts (at least within the English-speaking world) tend to focus on a white, middle-class experience of the condition. Being from a working-class family, I became keenly aware of this when I was caring for my dad.

There is some evidence that more nuanced stories are starting to be told that attempt to deal with the complexity, transformations and humanity associated with dementia, not simply the stereotypes of loss and obliteration so often portrayed. However, finding examples of more positive representations of people living with dementia is not easy. Even more sophisticated representations such as the novel and film *Still Alice* (Genova, 2012), which, as the title suggests, emphasises that Alice is still herself despite her dementia, portray the experience of dementia as one overwhelmingly of loss, and the diminishing of a person to something less than they were previously. Wendy Mitchell's autobiography *Somebody I Used to Know* takes a positive approach towards dementia as she writes about the new opportunities she has experienced, but alongside these, she also describes feeling as though she is losing her 'sense of self' and feeling 'powerless' (Mitchell, 2018, 284–5). There are also examples of novels where one of the main characters has dementia, although the story is not centred around the progression of their condition. *Elizabeth is Missing* (Healey, 2015) is one of the more thought-provoking examples of this as Maud, who has dementia, is the heroine who solves the mystery at the centre of the novel. She is the only person who has the crucial information, but she needs to find a way to communicate it. Overall, however, more nuanced examples are still few and far between. Given the overwhelmingly negative outlook of cultural representations of dementia, it is unfortunately questionable how far arts and media portrayals of the condition are helping to overcome the stigma around dementia at present.

What does this mean for libraries?

> Libraries are great spaces to bring the community together – they are a real community hub. It's where you go to learn – not only from a book, but also by sitting and talking to your neighbours. Libraries have the ability to build off connections and be a place where a person living with dementia feels comfortable and accepted as they go throughout their journey.
>
> (H. Cowie, e-mail to author, 9 June 2022)

As Heather Cowie from Dementia-Friendly Canada describes above, libraries are 'community hubs' that can be vital in supporting people with dementia and their carers to live well. A key concept used throughout this book is the notion of 'living well with dementia'. It is in contributing to 'living well' that libraries are likely to be able to make the greatest difference to the lives of people with dementia and their carers. 'Living well' means that a person with dementia can continue to live a positive and fulfilling life: enjoying interests they pursued before their diagnosis; participating in new activities; engaging in meaningful relationships; and feeling a sense of achievement and wellbeing. The idea that it is possible to live well with dementia is one that presents a challenge to many conventional views. The change in emphasis this approach requires is summed up by Tom Kitwood who argued, 'Our frame of reference should no longer be person-with-DEMENTIA, but PERSON-with-dementia' (Kitwood, 1997, 7).

The idea that a diagnosis of dementia is life-ending is deeply ingrained in many societies, but this is increasingly being challenged as new visions for living well with dementia emerge. The National Dementia Declaration for England sets out a series of quality outcomes, as described by people with dementia and their carers, that would indicate they were living well with dementia (DAA, 2010). These are discussed in greater detail in Chapter 2, but those which have particular relevance for library services are:

- I know that services are designed around me and my needs
- I have support that helps me live my life
- I have the knowledge and know-how to get what I need
- I live in an enabling and supportive environment where I feel valued and understood
- I have a sense of belonging and of being a valued part of family, community and civic life.

Despite the potential importance of libraries' role in supporting people with dementia and their carers, guidance from within the sector on how to go about this has been relatively limited. The International Federation of Library Associations and Institutions (IFLA) produced a set of *Guidelines for Library Services to Persons with Dementia* in 2007. However, this is badly in need of updating as it contains guidance that would now be widely criticised, such as referring to 'patients' and people 'suffering' from dementia, plus recommending children's picture books (which can be helpful in some circumstances but need to be used carefully – see Chapter 4). The American Library Association (ALA) provides some broad advice and links to best practice resources and guidance (ALA, 2020). In the UK, public library support for people with dementia is encompassed in the *Universal Health and Wellbeing Offer* (Libraries Connected, n.d.) which superseded a previous draft dementia-specific Universal Offer. Even though the latter, more detailed guide, is not currently in use, it is worth mentioning because it lists the following as aspects of the public library offer 'toolbox' for people with dementia and their carers: social and recreational activities; support groups; dementia-aware library staff; self-help dementia/carer book collections; reading programmes and promotions; range of formats including picture books; home library provision; care homes provision; dementia information and signposting service; and reminiscence-related materials.

Understandably, it can be tempting for libraries to want to argue that engagement with their services can help to reduce the risk of developing dementia or slow its development. However, it is important to be aware that, despite some interesting studies into the links between dementia and various types of cognitive or social stimulation – which are discussed in subsequent chapters – scientific evidence to support this is currently very limited. For instance, according to the WHO, although social activity has a wide range of other benefits to health and wellbeing, there is insufficient evidence to link social activity to a reduced risk of cognitive decline or dementia. The same review recommended that cognitive training may be offered to older adults with normal cognition and with mild cognitive impairment as, overall, the desirable effects of the intervention outweigh the undesirable effects. However, the quality of evidence to support a reduction in the risk of cognitive decline and/or dementia is very low to low (WHO, 2019).

Supporting people to live well with dementia

This book starts by asking the question, 'What is dementia?'. Chapter 1 presents an overview of the most common symptoms and types of dementia, with an emphasis on the fact that everyone is unique and dementia can affect people in many different ways. This chapter also introduces Kitwood's (1997) model of psychological needs and notion of personhood. An understanding of some of the basic theory frequently used amongst professionals caring for people with dementia is valuable when describing how library-based initiatives can contribute to approaches common within health and social care, thus helping library staff to gain buy-in from organisations beyond the library sector.

Chapter 2 sets the role of libraries within broader contexts, including the development of dementia-friendly and age-friendly communities. It describes ways in which library staff at all levels, but particularly those who are customer-facing, can support people with dementia and their carers. This chapter also discusses initiatives to support library staff who may be diagnosed with young-onset dementia and wish to continue working, or who are caring for someone with dementia.

Chapters 3, 4 and 5 offer a number of case studies illustrating ways in which libraries can support people with dementia and carers. These draw on varied contexts, including libraries from different sectors and locations and of different sizes. Chapter 3 focuses on library design and environments. It explores the ways in which the library space and environment can be organised with people with dementia in mind, for example, with regard to signage, colour schemes, layout, furniture and sensory spaces. Whilst some of the examples discussed are large-scale refurbishment or new-build projects, there are also ideas from smaller scale initiatives to make simple improvements to existing libraries. Chapter 4 looks at reading resources that libraries can offer; this includes resources about dementia, as well as materials for people with dementia and reading activities that are inclusive for people with dementia and their carers. This chapter focuses on three key ideas. The first is the ways in which dementia prompts us to widen what we might think of as 'texts' and expands our idea of 'reading' to include alternative types of resource. The second is the value of shared reading experiences. The final theme is the role of imagination in the lives of people with dementia. Chapter 5 considers further types of activity, in addition to reading, that might be offered within a library or as outreach provision. The case study examples described are divided into activities that support three areas: health and wellbeing; social interaction; and arts-based interventions.

Since the start of the COVID-19 pandemic, there have been significant changes in the ways in which libraries use technology. Chapter 6 discusses the potential role of technology in initiatives and activities for people with dementia and their carers, including the online delivery of activities and technology specifically designed to engage people with dementia, such as 'magic tables'.

Partnership working is often necessary to deliver the types of activities described in the previous chapters, so Chapter 7 considers examples of ways in which libraries can work in partnership with other organisations, including care homes, adult social care, arts organisations and community groups, to meet the needs of people with dementia and carers. It explores the challenges of partnership working and suggests some potential solutions.

Chapter 8 is about communications and marketing. This includes print materials but also digital communications. It explores considerations about terminology and language and reflects on broader design issues to be aware of, such as the layout of information and use of images.

It is important to involve people with dementia and their carers in the development of library services, as well as evaluating how well an intervention is working and adapting if necessary. Chapter 9 therefore discusses approaches that can be used in the evaluation and development of library services to ensure these activities are as inclusive as possible for people with dementia and their carers.

Finally, Chapter 10 concludes the book by exploring projected future trends in the incidence of dementia and the development of dementia care and reflects on the potential implications of these for libraries. It suggests key actions that are likely to be important for the ways in which libraries support people with dementia and their carers in the coming decades.

In the final section of the book, there is an annotated bibliography with links to useful resources and organisations.

Scope and terminology

The following is a brief note about some of the terminology used in this book. Of course, none of these terms are perfect and Chapter 8 discusses issues around language in greater detail. I have used terms that I feel work best overall for this book. When communicating with customers of particular libraries, there may be alternatives that are more appropriate for specific audiences.

Person with dementia or *person living with dementia* is used to indicate the person with the condition themselves.

Carer is used to refer to both people who provide unpaid care, such as a partner, family member or friend, and those who are employed to care for someone. In some quotes, alternative terms such as caregiver or care partner may be used depending on the terms used by an author or interviewee. In addition, in some situations the experiences of paid and unpaid carers are likely to differ, so distinctions are made between the two groups where it is important to reflect this.

People affected by dementia is used to include both people with dementia and carers.

While this book focuses on dementia, many of the approaches are also likely to be valuable for people living with related conditions, such as mild cognitive impairment (MCI) or Parkinson's disease, and in some cases also for a wider range of conditions, for example, autism.

This book is primarily aimed at library staff at all levels working across various sectors, including public libraries, health libraries, academic libraries, special libraries, prison libraries and school libraries, as well as information studies students and researchers. Hopefully, it will also be useful for professionals in other sectors, such as social care, health, museums and third sector organisations, who are interested in working more closely with libraries to support people with dementia and their carers.

1
What is Dementia?

> Treat me as I am. I am Jan or Pete or George. I've got dementia; I live well with dementia; and I'm putting a lot back into society.
> (Beth Johnson Foundation peer support group member)

This chapter provides a basic introduction to dementia. It focuses on the everyday impacts of living with dementia on both the person with the condition and their carers. It is important to stress that this book is not intended to provide detailed medical knowledge about dementia. There are useful resources listed in the annotated bibliography that go into greater detail about possible risk factors, symptoms, treatments and so forth should you require more information on these topics from reputable sources.

One of the difficulties of designing services for people living with dementia is that their symptoms, the ways in which their daily lives are affected and the types of support they need can vary hugely. Dementia is an umbrella term that includes a number of conditions, including Alzheimer's disease, vascular dementia and Lewy body dementia. The term 'dementia' describes a set of symptoms that often include memory loss and difficulties with thinking, problem-solving or language, as well as changes in mood and behaviour. The specific symptoms that people with dementia experience depend on which parts of the brain are affected and the underlying disease that is causing the dementia.

A person with dementia is likely to experience some of the following cognitive symptoms:

- changes in **day-to-day memory**, for example, recalling recent events
- difficulties **completing or initiating everyday tasks**, in particular planning, organising and decision-making

- issues with **communication**, for example, following a conversation or finding the right word
- challenges with **visuospatial skills**, such as judging distances
- problems with **orientation**, for example becoming confused about where they are, even in a familiar space.

They may also experience changes in mood or behaviour, for example becoming frustrated, apathetic, anxious, withdrawn or easily upset. With some types of dementia, people may experience hallucinations or delusions – strongly believing things that are not true. In the later stages of dementia in particular, people can experience physical symptoms such as weight loss and muscle weakness, as well changes in sleep patterns and appetite.

The conditions that cause dementia are usually progressive and symptoms get more severe over time. However, it is important to note that every experience of dementia is different – both in terms of the symptoms experienced and the rate of progression. In addition, while there is currently no cure for dementia, there is much that can be done to support people with dementia to live well.

This chapter starts by describing the most common types of dementia – Alzheimer's disease, vascular dementia, Lewy body dementia, frontotemporal dementia and mixed dementia – outlining the causes and most common symptoms of each. It also discusses young-onset dementia and mild cognitive impairment (MCI), before outlining typical stages someone with dementia is likely to experience. The complex ways in which dementia affects people make it difficult for those of us without the condition to imagine what it must be like to experience everyday life with dementia. This chapter also, therefore, describes some of the possible symptoms of dementia in detail and reflects on ways in which they might impact on people's use of library services. The chapter concludes by discussing the notion of person-centred care and explaining why this can be a helpful framework for libraries to use when considering the ways in which they offer services for people with dementia and their carers.

Types of dementia

As mentioned above, the term dementia is used to describe a number of different conditions that affect the brain. Whilst individuals are each affected differently, the descriptions below outline the most common symptoms displayed by people with particular types of dementia. The types of dementia described here are most prevalent, but there are also other, rarer, types of dementia, including Creutzfeldt-Jakob disease (CJD), HIV-associated neurocognitive disorder (HAND), Huntingdon's disease and corticobasal syndrome (CBS).

Alzheimer's disease

Alzheimer's disease is the most common form of dementia. There are more than 520,000 people with Alzheimer's disease in the UK (Alzheimer's Society, 2017a). The WHO estimates that Alzheimer's accounts for 60–70% of dementia cases worldwide, equating to between 33 and 38.5 million people based on 2021 figures (WHO, 2021). The changes in the brain involved in Alzheimer's disease are complex and still not fully understood. However, we do know that, in this form of dementia, proteins build up in the brain forming deposits called 'plaques' and 'tangles' that damage nerve cells and cause connections between them to be lost. Eventually, the nerve cells die and brain tissue is lost. Most people will develop some plaques and tangles in their brain as they age, but in people with Alzheimer's these are more numerous and usually begin in areas of the brain that are important for memory.

Because of the areas of the brain that tend to be affected first by Alzheimer's, short term memory problems are usually one of the first signs of the condition. Initially the symptoms are usually mild, but gradually, as more parts of the brain are damaged, symptoms get worse. For many people, the first signs of Alzheimer's include difficulty recalling recent events and learning new information. People with Alzheimer's may experience problems such as getting lost on a familiar journey or struggling to find the right word in a conversation. However, longer term memory is not usually affected in the early stages.

As the disease progresses, other symptoms are also likely to develop, including problems with thinking, reasoning, language and perception – for example, struggling to follow a conversation, making decisions, carrying out a sequence of tasks or judging distances. Some people with Alzheimer's may also experience changes in their mood, becoming anxious, depressed or easily annoyed, or may lose interest in talking to people or in taking part in interests and hobbies they previously enjoyed. However, whilst some skills may be lost, many are preserved for much longer periods because they are not controlled by the parts of the brain affected by the disease in the early stages. This is often especially true for skills learnt earlier in life: people with Alzheimer's may still be able to recite poems they learnt at school, for example. It is also worth noting that people are often able to recall the feelings (happiness, sadness, etc.) associated with a memory, even if they are not able to recall factual details of the experience.

In the later stages of Alzheimer's disease, a person's behaviour can change quite markedly. This might include being agitated, experiencing disturbed sleep patterns or acting aggressively. Some people experience delusions or hallucinations. However, it is worth considering that, whilst most of the literature about Alzheimer's discusses behaviours that are 'challenging', not all changes are necessarily negative. For instance, my dad experienced some loss of inhibition in the way that he talked to people compared to how he would have done previously, but this was often genuinely funny to both of us.

On average, a person will live between eight and ten years after the first symptoms of Alzheimer's disease appear. However, this varies considerably; some may live for around 20 years. It is therefore important to remember that someone with Alzheimer's may be living with the condition for a long time and it is only in the later stages that they are likely to experience severe symptoms (such as being less aware of what is happening around them) and have difficulties with basic activities (such as eating and walking). With the right support, people can often live well with Alzheimer's for many years.

Atypical Alzheimer's disease

For most people with Alzheimer's disease, their memory is affected first, but for some, memory problems are not the first symptom. This is referred to as atypical Alzheimer's and is more common in people diagnosed under the age of 65. Up to a third of people diagnosed with Alzheimer's under 65 have atypical Alzheimer's compared to just one in 20 of those over 65 (Alzheimer's Society, 2017a). The symptoms of atypical Alzheimer's vary depending on the part of the brain that is initially affected.

- *Frontal variant Alzheimer's disease.* In this type of Alzheimer's, symptoms are likely to include problems with planning and decision-making. The person may also behave in socially inappropriate ways or seem not to care about the feelings of others.
- *Logopenic progressive aphasia (LPA).* With this condition, there is damage to the part of the brain that produces speech, so the person may have problems finding the right word or need to take long pauses when speaking.
- *Posterior cortical atrophy (PCA).* In this type of dementia, there is damage to the part of the brain that processes information from the eyes, so symptoms are likely to include problems identifying objects or reading; struggling to judge distances; or appearing unco-ordinated (for example, when getting dressed).

Vascular dementia

Vascular dementia is the second most common type of dementia. There are around 150,000 people with vascular dementia in the UK (Alzheimer's Society, 2022). Vascular dementia alone accounts for around 10% of dementia cases, but exact numbers of people with this type of dementia are difficult to calculate as it is also often part of mixed dementia (see below). Vascular dementia is caused when there is reduced blood supply to the brain for some reason. If blood cannot reach the brain cells, for example, as the result of a stroke, the cells eventually die. This leads to problems with memory, thinking and reasoning. Vascular dementia is uncommon in people under the age of 65. Stroke, diabetes and heart disease all increase the risk of vascular dementia. Like other types of cardiovascular disease, vascular dementia is linked to high blood pressure, high cholesterol and being overweight.

There are several types of vascular dementia:

- *Post-stroke dementia*. A sudden disruption in blood supply to the brain as the result of a single large stroke starves the brain of oxygen and can lead to the death of brain tissue. About 20% of people who have a stroke go on to experience post-stroke dementia in the following six months.
- *Single-infarct* and *multi-infarct dementia*. These types of dementia are caused by a person experiencing one or more smaller strokes. Sometimes these are so small that the person does not even notice, but the disruption to blood supply leads to the death of a small area of brain tissue – an *infarct*. If this occurs in an important area of the brain, a single infarct can lead to dementia. More often, however, a person experiences a number of small strokes over a period of time that result in several infarcts that, together, lead to dementia.
- *Subcortical dementia*. This is caused by small vessel disease, which occurs when the blood vessels deep in the brain narrow, reducing blood flow.

Whereas a person with Alzheimer's disease tends to experience memory problems in the early stages, vascular dementia usually has different symptoms. These typically include:

- problems with planning, organising, decision-making or problem-solving
- difficulties following a series of steps or instructions
- slower speed of thought
- problems concentrating.

However, symptoms vary depending on the part(s) of the brain affected, and someone with vascular dementia may also experience problems with language, visuospatial skills and (usually mild) short term memory problems. They can also undergo mood changes, involving apathy, depression or anxiety say, or become prone to rapid mood swings.

With subcortical dementia, the person often experiences loss of bladder control and may become less steady on their feet and prone to falls. Other common symptoms of subcortical dementia include clumsiness, lack of facial expression and problems pronouncing words.

Stroke-related dementia often progresses in a 'stepped way', where the symptoms remain constant for a while, but then worsen suddenly if the person has another stroke. With subcortical dementia, on the other hand, symptoms usually worsen gradually.

Over time, someone with vascular dementia is likely to become increasingly confused or disorientated, and to experience more difficulties with reasoning and communication. Memory loss also occurs as the disease progresses. As with Alzheimer's disease, a person with vascular dementia may behave in ways that seem out of character; for example, becoming irritable, agitated or aggressive. Occasionally, they may experience delusions or hallucinations. As the condition progresses, someone with vascular dementia is likely to become increasingly frail and less aware of what is happening around them. On average, a person with vascular dementia lives for around five years after symptoms start, but this can vary greatly.

Lewy body dementia

Lewy body dementia accounts for around 10% to 15% of dementia cases (Dementia UK, 2022a). Lewy bodies are tiny clumps of protein that develop inside nerve cells. They contribute to lower levels of the chemicals that carry messages between nerve cells and a loss of connections between the nerve cells, which then die. Lewy bodies also cause Parkinson's disease along with other 'Lewy body disorders'. Because Lewy bodies cause a range of symptoms, some of which are shared by Alzheimer's disease and Parkinson's disease, especially in the early stages, Lewy body dementia is often wrongly diagnosed.

A person with Parkinson's disease is at high risk of going on to develop dementia; it is estimated that 50–80% of people with Parkinson's eventually experience dementia (Alzheimer's Association, 2022). When someone is diagnosed with Parkinson's at least a year *before* the symptoms of dementia develop, the condition is called Parkinson's disease dementia (PDD). Dementia with Lewy bodies (DLB) occurs when people experience symptoms of dementia without a previous diagnosis of Parkinson's. In these instances, it is often mistaken for Alzheimer's disease.

Lewy bodies can affect anywhere in the brain, leading to many different symptoms. The ways in which someone is affected will depend on what part(s) of the brain are involved. In broad terms, if the Lewy bodies are at the base of the brain, the person is likely to experience problems with movement. If the bodies are in the outer layers, the person is likely to experience problems with mental abilities. It is also possible for both mental and physical changes to happen at the same time. Typical features of Lewy body dementia include:

- varying levels of attention or alertness
- visual, and sometimes auditory, hallucinations
- movement problems (similar to Parkinson's disease)
- sleep disturbance – falling asleep during the day but being restless at night.

People with Lewy body dementia may also struggle to judge distances; see objects in three dimensions; and plan, organise and make decisions. They may also experience mood changes such as depression, agitation or aggression. Memory can be affected, but this may occur later and is often less affected compared to other types of dementia. Movement problems typically increase over time and a person with Lewy body dementia can experience falls and sometimes problems speaking or swallowing. On average, someone with Lewy body dementia lives for six to 12 years after the first symptoms, but, as with other types of dementia, this can vary considerably.

Frontotemporal dementia

Frontotemporal dementia (FTD), or Pick's disease, is a less common type of dementia than those discussed so far. It occurs when disease damages the frontal and temporal lobes in the brain. It is more likely to affect people under the age of 65. There are two main types of FTD that relate to the area of the brain that is affected first:

- *Behavioural variant FTD*. Damage to the frontal lobes causes changes in behaviour and personality and often the loss of inhibitions. A person with behavioural variant FTD may lose the motivation to do things they used to enjoy; struggle to focus on activities; find planning and decision-making difficult; lose the ability to understand what others might be feeling; over-eat or over-drink; or display repetitive or obsessive behaviours.
- *Primary progressive aphasia (PPA)*. Damage to the temporal lobes leads to difficulties with language (for example, finding the right word or having hesitant speech).

As the dementia progresses, the symptoms of the two types of FTD overlap; for example, someone with behavioural variant FTD is likely to go on to develop language problems over time, and vice versa. In the later stages, people with FTD usually experience muscle weakness and co-ordination problems. Unlike most types of dementia, there is often a family link in FTD diagnosis.

Mixed dementia

Around one in ten people with dementia have more than one type of disease. This is referred to as mixed dementia and is more often experienced by those aged over 75. The most common form of mixed dementia is Alzheimer's disease with vascular dementia, but other combinations are possible. Often, although a person has mixed dementia, one type is predominant. Symptoms will vary depending on the types of dementia present, but because there is more than one type of dementia, symptoms can be more noticeable and progress more rapidly. Because of the difficulties in diagnosing dementia, it is likely that some people diagnosed as having a single type of dementia may, in fact, have mixed dementia.

Young-onset dementia

Whilst the majority of people with dementia are older, in young-onset dementia, symptoms develop when the person is younger than 65. In the UK, an estimated 70,800 people were living with young-onset dementia in 2022. This accounts for approximately 7.5% of all people with dementia. The actual figure is likely to be higher because the average time to diagnosis is 4.4 years in younger people, double that for people aged over 65 (Dementia UK, 2022b).

As with dementia in older people, symptoms can vary considerably. Broadly, however, young people are less likely to experience memory problems, but are more likely to experience difficulties with movement, co-ordination or balance. People with Down's syndrome and some learning disabilities are more likely to develop young-onset dementia compared to the rest of the population.

In common with dementia amongst older people, Alzheimer's disease is the most common type of young-onset dementia. However, it is responsible for around a third of dementia diagnoses in younger people, compared to around two-thirds of older people with dementia. In addition, younger people are more likely to have atypical Alzheimer's than those in older age groups. FTD is also more common in younger people with dementia, as are some of the rarer types of dementia, such as CADASIL. Whilst it can affect younger people, young-onset dementia is most often diagnosed between the ages of 45 and 65.

Mild cognitive impairment

Mild cognitive impairment (MCI) is a condition in which someone has minor problems with cognition, such as memory or thinking. In MCI, the problems experienced are worse than would be expected for an average healthy person of the same age but are not significant enough to interfere greatly with daily life. It is estimated that between 5% and 20% of people over 65 have MCI (Alzheimer's Society, 2019a). Whilst MCI is not a type of dementia, people with this condition are more likely to go on to develop dementia. However, it is important to stress that not everyone with MCI will later develop dementia. Someone with MCI will have mild problems with one or more of the following: memory; reasoning, planning and problem-solving; attention; language; and visual depth perception. People with MCI may need some help with everyday tasks such as paying bills or managing medication.

Stages of dementia

As described above, the way in which dementia progresses varies considerably depending on the type of dementia, as well as from individual to individual. However, it can be helpful to think about the progression of dementia in three broad stages. This is especially useful when planning services and support for people with dementia as the types of support people are likely to require will vary at different stages.

Early-stage dementia

At this stage a person's symptoms are often relatively mild and not always easy to notice, especially by someone who does not know them well. In the early stages of dementia, people are able to remain largely independent, especially with the help of basic coping strategies, such as reminder lists, prompts and support with more complex tasks. Problems experienced at this stage can include memory problems (for example, not recalling recent events); difficulties planning and making more complex decisions; language and communication challenges (for example, struggling to find the right word); poor orientation (for example, getting lost even in a familiar place); visual-perceptual difficulties (for example, judging distance); and changes in mood or emotions.

Mid-stage dementia

At this stage the symptoms of dementia become more noticeable. For most people, this is the longest stage of dementia. Existing memory and thinking problems are likely to worsen (for example, remembering new information gets harder and the person may repeat the same question over and over). Language problems may also become more problematic (for example, it is harder to follow a conversation). Problems with orientation may become more severe too (for example, being confused even where they are at home). Some people with mid-stage dementia may also experience delusions and hallucinations. Noticeable behavioural changes most usually start at the mid-stage of dementia. These can include agitation, repetitive behaviour, disturbed sleep patterns and losing inhibitions.

Late-stage dementia

At this stage most people will need full-time care as the condition has a severe impact on many aspects of daily life. In the later stages the symptoms of all types of dementia become more similar. People may not recognise familiar objects or people and may experience time-shifting (see below). Delusions and hallucinations are more common. As language skills are reduced, people may respond more to sensory experiences, such as touch and listening to music. Physical difficulties also increase at this stage; these may include difficulties walking, eating, swallowing and incontinence.

Understanding dementia

There is no doubt that caring for someone with dementia can be challenging. The condition does not just impact on the person themselves, but also on their family members and friends. In part, the confusion, frustration and sadness family members can feel stems from the fact that dementia is so difficult to understand for someone who does not have it. This can also impact on the way in which people with dementia are treated within society more widely. Many of the most difficult aspects of living with dementia, such as stigma, isolation or frustration, are not inevitable symptoms of the condition itself, but result from the perceptions that society has of people with dementia. These perceptions and social attitudes can also mean that the task of taking care of a person with dementia becomes more challenging than it might otherwise be.

The complex ways in which dementia affects people make it difficult for those of us without the condition to imagine what it must be like to experience everyday life with dementia. We may feel we can partially relate to some symptoms, for example day-to-day memory loss, which, in its early stages, can seem like a more extreme version of something we all experience from time to time, such as forgetting someone's birthday or misplacing our car keys. However, dementia is much more complex than that and many of the symptoms can be difficult to immediately empathise with. The following section outlines some of the potential symptoms of dementia and explains why they may not, in fact, be as difficult to relate to as might first appear.

Time-shifting

People with dementia can experience time-shifting when the 'present' they feel themselves to be living in draws on aspects of the past. If a person with dementia has problems with short term memory, they may rely on older memories to make sense of their situation. This can mean, for instance, they do not understand more recent technology or do not recognise friends or family as they look now (expecting them to appear younger). A common example is someone trying to boil an electric kettle by putting it on the hob because they recall the activity of boiling a kettle from a time in their past, but not the newer process of using an electric kettle. Companies that provide resources specifically for people with dementia often 'disguise' new technology as older versions that people may more easily recognise, for example an MP3 player designed to resemble an old-fashioned wireless.

People with dementia often do not time-shift to the past in this way for long periods but can move in and out of different 'times' during the course of a day. Sometimes people who are retired will think they still go to work and will interpret what is going on around them in relation to this. For instance, my dad worked as a timekeeper at a steelworks, so would often think any piles of paper left around were time sheets he was working on.

Misperceptions

Misperceptions happen when the person with dementia sees one thing as something else. A common example is seeing a black door mat as a hole in the floor. Misperceptions can happen because of damage to the person's eyes or problems in another part of their visual system or brain. Sometimes misperceptions are caused by another condition rather than dementia itself; for example glaucoma or worsening eyesight due to ageing. However, whereas a person without dementia would realise that there is unlikely to be an actual hole in the doorway and can make sense of the misperception through knowing that they have vision problems, people with dementia may not always have that awareness, so instead try to make sense of a confusing situation in another way.

Misidentification

Misidentification is similar to misperception. It happens when someone has problems identifying specific objects or people, for example mistaking a mobile phone for a television remote, or confusing their son with their husband. Like misperceptions, misidentification can be the result of vision problems. However, it can also be linked to memory problems and time-shifting (see above). Like misperceptions, misidentification can be thought of as a way in which a person with dementia is trying to make sense of the world. For instance, someone may not remember that she has children, so assumes a man who is familiar and she feels affection for is her husband – especially if her son looks like his father did when he was younger.

Delusions

Delusions are strongly held, but false, beliefs that can make someone feel suspicious of those around them and feel threatened when there is no real reason to feel that way. The person may over-react to innocent or minor incidents and jump to conclusions with little evidence, for example thinking a neighbour is watching them when they are simply waiting for a delivery. Common delusions experienced by people with dementia include the following:

- *Theft – thinking something has been stolen because they cannot find it.* This can be linked to memory problems, as someone with dementia makes sense of having forgotten where they left something by thinking it was stolen. This type of delusion can lead people to 'hide' things in unusual places, away from potential 'thieves'.
- *Believing those close to them are trying to harm them in some way.* This might be linked to misidentification (see above); for example, they may not recognise a friend who visits them and think there is a stranger in their home.
- *Not believing their home is their real home.* This can particularly be the case for a home they have only lived in in the recent past (or has been altered to better suit their physical needs) and so seems unfamiliar (see time-shifting above).

Language and communication

People living with dementia can experience a range of language and communication problems. These may include:

- having trouble finding the right words
- using a related or substitute word (for example, asking for 'milk' when they want a cup of tea)
- repeating words or phrases
- describing something rather than naming it (for example, a 'thing for writing' rather than a pen)
- using words that have no obvious meaning in a particular context
- going back to their first language (if they learnt an additional language that they used regularly at a later point in their life)
- having difficulty recognising other people's emotions in conversations (for example, when someone is being humorous)
- having problems following a conversation, especially one in a noisy environment or with several speakers involved.

Understandably, not being able to communicate as they used to can be frustrating. Like other symptoms of dementia, language problems can vary from day-to-day or at different times of the day.

Restlessness

Some people with dementia may regularly walk about, seemingly without an obvious purpose – this might be walking around their home, but also leaving their house (and then perhaps finding it difficult to find their way back because of memory and orientation problems). The person may not be able to explain why they are walking, so finding the underlying reason can be challenging. Common reasons for walking about include:

- starting out with a purpose, but then forgetting where they intended to go due to short term memory problems
- confusion about the time of day (for example, thinking it is morning and they need to get up when it is still the middle of the night)
- searching for someone or something from the past (for example, someone they used to live with)
- trying to relieve pain or discomfort
- feeling anxious, agitated or bored
- feeling 'lost' in an unfamiliar environment.

Whilst this section has provided information about some common dementia symptoms, a powerful way of engaging with and understanding the issues faced by people with dementia is to 'walk the patch'. This means spending time with people with dementia in their home or anywhere else that they may want to go to, for example in shops, leisure centres or on public transport, as well as in libraries. Seeing the world through the eyes of someone experiencing dementia can be a revelatory experience. There are films and apps that attempt to show this (see the annotated bibliography for examples). An example is *Drawing from our Experience: Stories of travelling with dementia* (Hyde et al., 2019), which was co-created by artists and people living with dementia who spent a day travelling together from Dundee railway station in Scotland to the city centre and an art gallery. The group then produced a comic that portrayed their experiences to help those without the condition to understand better what it is like to navigate the world with dementia and to appreciate how people in customer service roles can make journeys easier.

Potential impacts on the use of library services

So far, this chapter has outlined the main ways in which people with dementia are likely to be affected by their condition, but what does this mean in practice for library services? Despite the fact that most people live with dementia for a number of years, many find it difficult to negotiate public spaces and environments, meaning access to social groups or cultural activities, including libraries, is trickier. This can lead to a further sense of isolation for both the person with dementia and their carers, who often find their opportunities to access social and cultural opportunities reduced too. Some of the main ways in which dementia may impact people's use of library services include the following:

- access to the library building – including signposting, accessibility of the building and using public transport to get there if they need to
- orientation within the library space – such as signage, finding what they are looking for, knowing how/who to ask for help
- understanding how to use features of the library – for instance, using a self-issue machine or an online catalogue rather than a card catalogue that they may recall from the past
- planning and memory skills – for instance, remembering to attend activities or to return books by their due date
- communication issues – challenges in communicating with library staff and other customers, as well as changes in reading skills.

For carers, there can also be the worry, possibly based on a more traditional image of libraries, that the person with dementia may behave in ways that are considered 'inappropriate' in a library, leading to adverse reactions from other customers or staff. These various challenges, and ways of addressing them, are explored in detail in the subsequent chapters of this book.

Person-centred care

There are a number of approaches to dementia care: some have a more medical emphasis, whilst others focus on the social aspects of living with dementia. As a non-medical service, it makes sense that libraries have a more obvious social or wellbeing role to play in supporting people with dementia and their carers. This book is therefore centred around the notion of person-centred care, an approach that is commonly used in health and social care services in the UK and elsewhere. Person-centred care is care and support that is tailored around an individual's needs, preferences, values, beliefs, life history and other things that are important to a person. It puts the person first and avoids a person with dementia being 'reduced to their illness'. Dawn Brooker (2004) outlines four essential elements of person-centred dementia care:

1 Valuing people with dementia and those who care for them: promoting their citizenship rights and entitlements.
2 Treating people as individuals: appreciating their unique history and personality and considering how these influence their dementia.
3 Looking at the world from the perspective of the person with dementia.
4 Recognising the importance of relationships and interactions with others to the person living with dementia and their potential for promoting wellbeing.

This approach to dementia care aims to help maintain an individual's 'personhood' by focusing on their identity, needs and values. 'Personhood' or 'self' is a complex concept. Tom Kitwood defined personhood as 'a standing or status that is bestowed upon one human being, by others, in the context of relationship and social being. It implies recognition, respect and trust' (Kitwood, 1997, 8). It recognises that every person is unique, with distinct needs, preferences, values and life history, and that these make up their unique identity. However, it is important to remember that none of us is a single, fixed personality and many of the characteristics that make up our 'personhood' may change over time and in different circumstances. People – and especially those with dementia – are not 'frozen' in time but recognised as having the potential for changing interests, opinions and preferences.

When a person with dementia becomes less able to take part in certain activities, or experiences increasing problems interacting and communicating with other people, ways of supporting the person to maintain their sense of personhood need to be identified. In the 1990s, Kitwood strongly advocated respect for personhood in dementia care and its key role in promoting quality of life. He claimed awareness of personhood is so fundamental to quality of life that it can deliver better quality of life outcomes in care settings than medical interventions alone. As well as the obvious neurological impairment experienced, Kitwood argued that a person's experience of dementia is also affected by their biography, personality, broader physical health and their social environment. According to Kitwood, the interactions of others are extremely significant in sustaining, or alternatively undermining, personhood. Poor social interactions and social isolation can undermine a person's position with others, leaving them unable to assert their identity and struggling to maintain their sense of personhood (Kitwood, 1997).

Developing this idea into practical actions, Kitwood (1997) looked at what people with dementia need from those around them to enable them to exist as a person. He chose to represent these needs as a flower with love at the centre surrounded five 'petals' – comfort, attachment, inclusion, occupation and identity:

1 **Comfort** is the provision of warmth and closeness to others to provide security and relaxation and to decrease anxiety. Comfort can be provided physically, but also through words and gestures.
2 **Attachment** is about bonding, connection, nurture, trust and relationships. It means knowing you have people you can turn to in times of need.
3 **Inclusion** is about being in the social world and being welcomed and accepted as part of a group. It means recognising a person's worth and including them in discussions or activities.
4 **Occupation** relates to being involved in an activity that is personally meaningful, and feeling you have control over what happens and how it is done.
5 **Identity** relates to knowing who you are and having a sense of continuity with the past, for example through celebrating a person's life story. Identity is bolstered by being surrounded by people who know about you and hold you in esteem.

This simple model offers a way to explore the impact of library services and activities for people with dementia and their carers. Of course, not every activity will address all five needs, but each intervention intended to support the needs of people with dementia should contribute to at least one aspect. For this reason, several of the case studies included in later chapters of this book are described in terms of the needs they address. This can help library staff to identify where they are potentially making an impact on the lives of people with dementia and can also help them to describe interventions using concepts that are likely to be familiar to professionals from other sectors, such as health and social care.

Importantly, Tom Kitwood argued that the progression of dementia should not necessarily be seen as a downward trajectory and that, through good communication, which he calls 'positive person work', a person's overall life experience may improve despite the physical progression of their dementia. Dawn Brooker (2007) developed this idea further to identify 17 'personal enhancers' that describe positive ways of interacting with a person with dementia:

1. Warmth: demonstrating genuine affection, care and concern.
2. Holding: providing safety, security and comfort.
3. Relaxed pace: creating a relaxed atmosphere and letting the person with dementia set the pace.
4. Respect: valuing the person with dementia and recognising their experience.
5. Acceptance: having an attitude of acceptance or positive regard for the person with dementia.
6. Celebration: recognising and taking delight in a person's skills and achievements.
7. Acknowledgement: recognising, accepting and valuing the person as a unique individual.
8. Genuineness: being open and honest, but in a way that is sensitive to a person's needs and feelings.
9. Validation: recognising and supporting the person's reality.
10. Empowerment: assisting the person with dementia to discover or use their skills and abilities.
11. Facilitation: assessing the level of support required and providing it.
12. Enabling: recognising and encouraging a person's level of engagement.
13. Collaboration: treating the person with dementia as a full and equal partner in what is happening.
14. Recognition: accepting the person's uniqueness with an open attitude.
15. Including: enabling and encouraging the person to feel included.
16. Belonging: providing a sense of acceptance.
17. Fun: supporting a free, creative way of being, using fun and humour.

The following are just a few examples of how these ideas might take place in a library environment:

- When reading with someone, ask if they want to read along with you, then maybe encourage them to read alone if they seem confident (empowerment, enabling).
- If someone asks for help finding a book that seems unusual for their age or other circumstances, help them to find it rather than guiding them to something you feel is more suitable (acceptance, acknowledgement).
- If you are running an activity for people with dementia, do not feel you need to rush people to get through everything you had planned. Let the group set the pace; you can come back to anything you do not have time for in another session (relaxed pace, collaboration).
- Listen carefully, respond to and encourage memories shared by someone in a reminiscence session, even if you think these may not be factually accurate (respect, validation).

The notion of person-centred care is now widely accepted as a framework for dementia care in several countries. For example, in the UK, NICE (National Institute for Health and Care Excellence) guidelines, which are intended to improve outcomes for people using the NHS and other public health and social care services, are based around person-centred care. They recommend involving people living with dementia in decisions about their care and emphasise the importance of assessing the likes, dislikes, routines and personal history of a person living with dementia (NICE, 2018). The basic principles of person-centred care should, therefore, be familiar to those working within health and social care in the UK. Guidance with a similar emphasis has been published in other countries too.

In Australia, the *Aged Care Quality Standards* (Aged Care Quality and Safety Commission, 2021) encourage providers to offer person-centred (or consumer-centred) care across all care settings. These Standards have been designed to directly focus on how person-centred care should be delivered by providers. In Canada, *A Dementia Strategy for Canada: Together We Aspire* (Public Health Agency of Canada, 2019) also sets out the government's aspirations for more person-centred approaches to dementia care. This approach is not limited to the English-speaking world; Chile's *National Dementia Plan*, for example, recommends a health model 'where people are understood in their entirety and through their individual history, being part of a system where respect, dignity and solidarity enable the building of a compassionate society' [author translation] (Ministerio de Salud, 2017).

Another important development linked to the notion of person-centred care is the increasing awareness of the value of creative arts practice in dementia (SCIE, 2020b). Active engagement in the arts has been found to have the power to transform the lives of people with dementia through greater fulfilment, confidence, skills development, desire to socialise and the relief of stress. The creative, imaginative and emotional parts of a person with dementia often remain relatively strong, despite the condition's negative effects on their cognitive abilities. Libraries obviously have a potential role to play in supporting creative arts activities involving people with dementia and this is discussed in greater detail in Chapters 4 and 5.

Conclusions

This chapter has outlined some of the common symptoms of dementia and reflected on how these might impact on a person's daily life. There is currently no cure for dementia and limited treatment options. This makes the role of community organisations, such as libraries, especially important in making it as easy as possible for people with dementia to live positive, fulfilling lives. Chapter 2 looks in more detail at the ways in which libraries can support people living with dementia and their carers.

2
Supporting People Living with Dementia and their Carers

> It strikes me that it's just the little things . . . . People ask, 'What's the big, innovative thing I can do?' But really, it's about communication strategies.
> (Heather Cowie, National Project Manager, Dementia-Friendly Canada, in conversation with author)

Living with dementia has a major impact on people's lives – and the lives of those who care for them. This book focuses on ways in which libraries can support people to live well with dementia, but what does this actually mean? A wide range of factors can be thought of as contributing to a good life. According to Age UK, these can be broadly grouped under the following headings: personal wellbeing, positive relationships and active daily lives (Jopling, 2017).

As well as being difficult to pin down, the notion of 'living well' is highly individual. The National Dementia Declaration for England has laid out seven quality outcomes, as described by people with dementia and their carers that indicate they are living well with dementia (DAA, 2010). These are:

1 I have personal choice and control or influence over decisions about me.
2 I know that services are designed around me and my needs.
3 I have support that helps me live my life.
4 I have the knowledge and know-how to get what I need.
5 I live in an enabling and supportive environment where I feel valued and understood.
6 I have a sense of belonging and of being a valued part of family, community and civic life.
7 I know there is research going on which delivers a better life for me now and hope for the future.

However, in practice people with dementia often find it challenging to continue with activities they enjoyed previously. A survey by the UK Alzheimer's Society found that:

- 35% of people with dementia said that they only go out once a week or less, and 10% once a month or less
- people said that they had to give up activities such as getting out of the house (28%), shopping (23%), exercise (22%) and using transport (16%)
- 9% of people with dementia said they had had to stop doing *all* the things they used to do
- 63% of people with dementia did not want to try new things. (Green and Lakey, 2013)

These are worrying statistics. In some instances, it is aspects of dementia itself that prevents people from doing the things they used to, for example having to give up driving because of visuospatial problems. More often, however, it is not their condition in itself that prevents people continuing with the activities they took part in previously; rather, it is the fact that the communities and environments they interact with lack the support for people with dementia that would allow them to continue to live their everyday lives. This chapter starts by setting dementia within the context of a social model of disability and rights-based approaches that are useful in informing community responses to dementia. It then looks specifically at the creation of dementia-friendly communities and how libraries as community-focused organisations can play an important role in their development. The remainder of the chapter focuses on the role that individual library staff can play on a day-to-day basis in supporting both customers and colleagues with dementia or those who are carers. It concludes by outlining some of the types of training opportunities available to library staff who wish to develop their skills in supporting people with dementia.

Social model of disability

The social model of disability provides a way of thinking about the needs of people with dementia and their carers that can be helpful in finding approaches to allow them to continue to take part in everyday activities. In a medical model of disability, it is a person's condition that is responsible for the difficulties they experience; for example, a wheelchair user cannot catch a train because they are unable get up the step to enter the carriage. In contrast, the social model of disability argues that people are not impaired by their condition but as a result of social, economic, attitudinal, physical, architectural or environmental factors. So, looking at the same problem using this model, a wheelchair user is unable to board a train because of the way that stations and trains have been designed (Campaign for Level Boarding, n.d.).

It needs to be acknowledged that dementia is not always recognised as a disability. However, as the UK All Party Parliamentary Group (APPG) on Dementia (2019) pointed out, dementia is a disability under both UK law and international convention, specifically the UN *Convention on the Rights of Persons with Disabilities* (CRPD) (UN DESA, 2022). Almost all those surveyed as part of this parliamentary inquiry thought that people with dementia are treated differently to people with other health conditions or disabilities – possibly due to the 'hidden' nature of dementia and stigma surrounding the condition. Whilst some people with dementia may feel labelling the condition as a disability has negative connotations, the recognition of dementia as a disability can help people with dementia and their carers to ensure their rights are protected in relation to employment, transport, housing and other areas. In particular, in relation to community life the UK APPG on Dementia recommended that 'communities must increase their awareness and understanding of dementia and people need to be supported through the development of inclusive communities where no one is excluded or has to face dementia alone' (APPG on Dementia, 2019, 7).

Rights-based approaches

One means through which the notion of living well with dementia can be put into practice is through right-based approaches. Rights-based approaches are an important component of the social model of disability and can be effective in supporting the development of services that enable people to live well. They do this by helping to shift emphasis away from 'managing' people with dementia towards enabling them to live the lives they choose, and away from the 'deficits' associated with dementia towards breaking down the barriers experienced by people living with the condition. Understanding dementia through the frame of disability rights helps to widen the scope of services and systems that need to be part of a community's response to dementia and creates an impetus for action.

A series of Dementia Statements developed by the Dementia Action Alliance in the UK, in consultation with people affected by dementia and other key stakeholders, state:

- We have the right to be recognised as who we are, to make choices about our lives including taking risks, and to contribute to society. Our diagnosis should not define us, nor should we be ashamed of it.

- We have the right to continue with day-to-day and family life, without discrimination or unfair cost, to be accepted and included in our communities and not live in isolation or loneliness.
- We have the right to an early and accurate diagnosis, and to receive evidence-based, appropriate, compassionate and properly funded care and treatment, from trained people who understand us and how dementia affects us. This must meet our needs, wherever we live.
- We have the right to be respected, and recognised as partners in care, provided with education, support, services and training which enables us to plan and make decisions about the future.
- We have the right to know about and decide if we want to be involved in research that looks at cause, cure and care for dementia and be supported to take part. (DAA, 2017)

Dementia-friendly communities

Part of implementing a social model of disability in relation to dementia involves not just providing services, activities and opportunities specifically for people with dementia, but also ensuring that mainstream provision is as accessible as possible. Often, people with dementia want to maintain their everyday activities, rather than being channelled into (or potentially 'hidden away' in) 'specialist' provision. Many people with dementia feel that the support they need to participate in their community and to do the everyday things they want to do, for example shopping, socialising or using public transport, is not available. As a result, many do not feel that they are a part of their local communities. The creation of dementia-friendly, or dementia-inclusive, communities is an attempt to meet this need.

The UK Alzheimer's Society defines a dementia-friendly community as, 'one in which people with dementia are empowered to have high aspirations and feel confident, knowing they can contribute and participate in activities that are meaningful to them' (Green and Lakey, 2013, viii). In more practical terms, a dementia-friendly community enables people with dementia to find their way around and be safe; access local facilities such as banks, shops, cafes, libraries and post offices; and maintain their social networks so they feel they continue to belong.

Focusing in on how this might apply within individual organisations, the Alzheimer Society of Saskatchewan in Canada (2019) describes a dementia-friendly business as one that:

- considers that a person with dementia may experience the world differently and incorporates this knowledge accordingly when making decisions that affect policy or design
- is responsive to the needs of people affected by dementia and makes efforts to understand the impact of dementia in their community by ensuring that people living with dementia and their care partners are included and consulted in conversations about becoming dementia friendly
- actively works to challenge stigma by creating a culture of openness about dementia, by addressing misconceptions and promoting evidence-based information and awareness
- addresses barriers in the physical environment to provide a more accessible, accommodating and welcoming space.

Being dementia friendly is, therefore, not only about ensuring spaces and services meet the needs of people with dementia, but also about ensuring people with dementia feel included and addressing the stigma around dementia. Dementia-friendly communities can help to tackle the stigma and social isolation associated with the condition through strategies to engage and include people with dementia in community life. The availability of accessible community activities that are appropriate to the needs of people living with dementia, along with suitable transport options, are important for a community to become dementia friendly. The engagement of people living with dementia, not only through specialised provision but also in mainstream community activities, is also important.

The creation of dementia-friendly communities has the potential to change the way we think about living with dementia. It means a shift in focus from simply meeting the immediate physical and health needs of a person to a more holistic approach that supports the person to achieve the best quality of life reasonably possible. Dementia-friendly communities have the potential to reduce stigma and increase understanding through greater awareness, as well as recognising the rights and capabilities of people with dementia so that they feel respected and involved in decisions about their lives.

The ultimate aim is to create a society where dementia is 'normalised' and people with dementia are supported to live fulfilling lives. It is also worth drawing attention to another concept, perhaps less frequently used – 'dementia positive'. This term emphasises the importance of not only taking care of and respecting people with dementia, but also seeing them as equal contributors to society. So, in the case of libraries, this might mean moving beyond staff training, dementia-friendly building design and the provision of resources and activities, to initiatives that draw on the strengths of people with dementia and provide opportunities for them to contribute to collection development, for example. (See Chapter 5 for examples.)

In 2013 the UK Alzheimer's Society launched a recognition process for dementia-friendly communities that outlined ten characteristics. This suggested that becoming dementia friendly means:

1. Shaping communities around the views of people with dementia and their carers.
2. Challenging stigma and building awareness.
3. Ensuring that activities include people with dementia.
4. Empowering people with dementia and recognising their contribution.
5. Befrienders helping people with dementia engage in community life.
6. Maintaining independence by delivering community-based solutions.
7. Easy to navigate physical environments.
8. Businesses and services that respond to customers with dementia.
9. Ensuring early diagnosis, personalised and integrated care is the norm.
10. Appropriate transport. (Green and Lakey, 2013)

Once a community has demonstrated how they meet these criteria, they are issued with a symbol that they can give to organisations and businesses in their community that wish to be part of the dementia-friendly communities initiative and have outlined their actions towards becoming dementia friendly.

Initiatives that can help to achieve dementia-friendly community status that may be particularly relevant to libraries include:

- collaborations with local community organisations to support the continued involvement of people with dementia in community activities
- a physical environment that supports the needs of people living with dementia (for example, in the design of pathways, signage and lighting)
- showcasing stories of people with dementia volunteering within the community
- programmes to support people with dementia to remain in employment. (ADI, 2016)

It is important to remember that people with dementia and carers from different communities, whether these are defined by geographical area or by cultural or social groupings, often face very different challenges. The experiences of people with dementia in the local community should be at the forefront of any dementia-friendly community programme. Dementia-friendly communities should be shaped by the needs and opinions of people living with dementia *within that community*, together with input from carers. In addition to dementia-friendly initiatives, it is also important to acknowledge the value of age-friendly communities as these often have a lot of overlap. However, age-friendly communities do not necessarily address the specific needs of people with dementia and, as they are focused on older people, may not include the needs of people with young-onset dementia.

Case study: Alzheimer Society of Saskatchewan – Dementia Friendly Toolkit for Libraries

The Alzheimer Society of Saskatchewan in Canada has developed a Dementia Friendly Communities initiative to assist communities of all types and sizes to become more dementia friendly. Their vision is that communities will recognise that a person with dementia may experience the world differently and will be prepared to make a conscious effort to reduce stigma and become more supportive, inclusive and accessible. The Dementia Friendly Communities initiative seeks to promote the number of locally based supports; strengthen community relationships; increase awareness and understanding; and assist communities to address the social and physical barriers that can make inclusion challenging for those affected by dementia. As part of this initiative, the Alzheimer Society of Saskatchewan has produced a Library Edition of their Dementia Friendly Toolkit. This includes advice on staffing; physical environments; and practices and programmes, as well as practical steps to help libraries to become more dementia friendly, including tip sheets and checklists specifically for libraries (Alzheimer Society of Saskatchewan, 2019).

Abby Wolfe, Public Awareness Co-ordinator at the Alzheimer Society of Saskatchewan, describes the process of developing the toolkit and why they were keen to work with libraries specifically as a key organisation in the development of dementia-friendly communities:

> We did some focus groups with individuals with lived experience of dementia. We invited them to have a conversation about what a dementia-friendly community might look like and what that might mean. What we heard from them was that the community really does make a difference in terms of those daily places that they used to be familiar going to and that they want to keep as part of their routine. In those focus groups, people talked about things like post offices or grocery stores or libraries. And we really took that to heart and focused on the fact that when we're talking about a dementia-friendly community, it's actually about the places that people experience in their daily lives. In Saskatchewan, we have quite a broad geographical spread – a low population density and a large size of province. The considerations that we had were around how we can find the sector that will best leverage uptake in rural areas and remote areas of the province, as well as urban areas. Libraries started to really become the sector that stuck out to us, because in small places they often serve as the community hubs where folks are already going to access services. Maybe they're already going to the library to have internet connection, especially in those rural and remote areas, and they're already seeing the library as a site of interaction.

> We knew that libraries had potential then to really be a place that could make a difference in reducing social isolation and could start to strengthen the supports and connections that folks have in the community. The other aspect of that was that libraries really have the power to create positive outcomes for both folks living with dementia and care partners, because some of the care partners that participated in our focus groups or that shared feedback with our programmes and services teams talked about how they experience some losses and changes in routine and an increase in social isolation when those care needs increased.
>
> So those were all reasons that, for us, libraries just started to be that shining example of a really great opportunity to connect. Those focus groups helped us lay the foundation of how to talk with libraries about dementia, how to tie in that alignment between their efforts to be inclusive and supportive organisations for members of the public and our efforts to help people affected by dementia remain meaningfully engaged in their communities. So, that forms the basis of the Library Edition of the toolkit and in April 2019 we released it at the provincial Saskatchewan Library Association Conference.
>
> (A. Wolfe, conversation with author, 15 November 2021)

Supporting library customers with dementia and their carers

As organisations, libraries have a potentially crucial role to play within their localities as part of the creation of dementia-friendly communities, but what does this mean for individual library staff and the ways in which they interact with customers with dementia and carers? Of course, thoughtful and helpful service can make a big difference to anyone who is feeling vulnerable. People with dementia have said that more care and support would enable them to do more in their local area and undertake everyday tasks and activities (Alzheimer's Society, 2015a). As individuals within their local community that people with dementia are likely to have regular contact with, customer-facing library staff are in a critical position to influence the everyday experience of a person with dementia.

The common symptoms of dementia such as memory loss and problems with communication, thinking and reasoning might well affect how somebody with dementia interacts with other people. They may find it hard to remember recent conversations and events, so they may not recall a conversation you had last week or even a few minutes ago. They may not remember someone's name or recognise them, even if they have known them for many years. If someone with dementia is finding it difficult to process information or is feeling disoriented, they may not be able to answer what appear to be simple questions or take in what you are saying. Busy environments can make it especially difficult for someone with dementia to concentrate on a conversation. Furthermore, they may not remember what they were doing or intending to do, forget where they left something or have difficulty finding their way around – even in a building they have been visiting for a long time.

Whilst displaying the types of behaviours described above *might* indicate that someone has dementia, the fact that there are no obvious physical signs of the condition means that determining whether or not a library customer actually has dementia can be difficult. Some libraries, along with other businesses and organisations, take part in the sunflower lanyard scheme for people with non-visible disabilities. The intention of this scheme is to allow someone with a hidden disability, such as autism, dementia or chronic pain, to signal discreetly to staff that the wearer (or someone with them) may need more time and support. Many people have found this scheme extremely helpful. However, others have expressed concerns because they do not want to disclose their condition or have concerns about vulnerable people becoming more identifiable. Another factor to be aware of is that the lanyard scheme covers a wide range of disabilities, so it does not indicate what type of support someone might find useful, which can obviously vary tremendously. The issue of identifying a customer with dementia is further complicated by the fact that more than half of people who have dementia have not received a diagnosis (SCIE, 2020a). Consequently, you may well not be sure whether a customer has dementia and, indeed, they may not always be aware themselves.

Ultimately, however, whether a customer has dementia or not does not really matter; what is important is that you are supporting them in a way that best meets their individual needs. Consequently, the advice below may be useful when interacting with any customers who display symptoms that suggest it is possible they may have dementia. A number of these tips will probably be familiar – or obvious – to library staff as they are basic principles of good customer service.

Tips for communicating with someone with dementia

Of course everyone is different, but the following suggestions may be helpful when communicating with a person with dementia – and often with other customers too:

1 Try to make sure you are somewhere quiet and calm, with good lighting. For example, if the area around the issue desk is busy or noisy, you might ask someone if they're happy to move to a different area of the library to have a conversation.
2 Stand or sit where the person can see and hear you as clearly as possible – usually this will be in front of them, at eye-level and with your face well-lit.

3. Listen carefully to what the person is saying. Offer encouragement both verbally and non-verbally, for example, by making eye contact and nodding.
4. If you have not fully understood what the person has said, ask them to repeat it. If you are still unclear, rephrase their answer to check your understanding of what they meant.
5. Allow the person plenty of time to respond – it may take them a little longer to process the information and work out their response.
6. Try not to interrupt the person or to be too quick to assume you know what they are trying to say.
7. Try not to appear to be rushed, stressed or impatient. Try to make sure your body language is open and relaxed. Avoid speaking sharply or raising your voice.
8. Make sure that your body language and facial expression match what you are saying, even if this feels a bit forced.
9. If the person is struggling to follow you, go at a slightly slower pace than usual; use short, simple sentences; and avoid asking complicated questions or using 'library jargon'.
10. Stick to one idea at a time. Giving someone a choice is important, but too many options can be confusing and frustrating. Some advice recommends focusing on closed 'yes/no' questions: this approach can sometimes be helpful but take care that you are not limiting a person's options or opportunities to express themselves by doing this.
11. If the person does not seem to understand what you are saying, even after you repeat it, try saying it in a slightly different way instead.
12. If the person does not appear to understand a particular word you are using, try using prompts, props and context to help with naming items. The person may recognise an object and what it is used for, even if they cannot remember what it is called.
13. If the person repeats a question, it will not help to tell them that they have heard the information before. Give simple answers and repeat them as necessary. In some cases, it can be helpful to write the answer down so that the person has a note of it.
14. If a person with dementia is accompanied by a carer, continue to involve the person with dementia directly in the conversation, rather than only focusing on the person they are with.
15. It is fine to laugh together about misunderstandings and mistakes, but make sure the person does not feel you are laughing at them.

Many organisations provide advice on communicating with people with dementia. Some links and resources are included in the annotated bibliography. However, it is important to consider to what extent this general guidance applies within your own local context or to individuals you are communicating with. For example, the UK Alzheimer's Society's guidance says that 'Words like "love", "honey" and "dear" can be patronising for people living with dementia' (Alzheimer's Society, 2018). However, whilst that might be true in some communities, where I live in the north of England, calling someone 'love' – or a similar term – is a part of everyday conversation, including in customer service situations. For many people, *not* calling a person with dementia 'love' would single them out and mean treating them differently to other customers.

Tips for offering support to someone with dementia using the library

Whilst the above tips are applicable in any situation when you are trying to support or communicate with someone with dementia, there may be times when someone wants to carry out a specific activity in a library. The following are some ideas for ways to support them in this context.

1. If someone cannot remember how to do something, such as how to find a particular book, offer to show them how to do it. However, as much as possible, do the task *with* them not *for* them.
2. Somebody with dementia may feel anxious about their ability to carry out tasks or activities, such as logging onto the library Wi-Fi. Try not to put them under pressure: break down the activity into smaller tasks, supporting them along the way.
3. If someone appears to be looking for something, approach them face-on and ask if you can help. Do not call out from across the library. If they want something in another part of the library, offer to go with them to show them where it is rather than simply giving directions, which they may not remember or find difficult to follow.
4. People with dementia may have problems with money or their payment card, for example if they want to pay for photocopying at the library. Be patient: tell them there is no hurry and ask if you can help counting out the right money.
5. If someone cannot remember significant information, for example their PIN for self-issue or where they have put their library card, make sure you are aware of your organisation's alternative procedures that will help them access the service or information they require (for example, issuing books manually).

Some libraries offer special membership cards for people with dementia with features such as access to additional audio or non-print materials, extended loan periods and no fines for overdue items. Libraries often also have special library cards for carers that allow them to borrow items for longer, avoid fines and make requests for free.

Finally, it is important to remember that, like all of us, people with dementia will have 'good days' and 'bad days'. The difference is that most of us can cover up when we are having a bad day and act more positive than we feel. Someone with dementia may be less likely to be able to do this. If a person with dementia is having a bad day, they may be less willing to join in an activity they usually enjoy or may require more support doing something. On a good day, the amount or type of support they need or the way they interact may well be different again.

Support for carers

Much of this chapter has focused on support for people with dementia. However, it is important to consider that, as research has shown, overall, carers are usually much less positive about the state of their relationships than people with dementia themselves (Jopling, 2017). Potential challenges presented by caring for someone with dementia include: changing roles (for example, spouses taking on tasks that the other person used to do or child/parent role reversal); a sense of guilt about the perceived burden on the carer; a need for time away from the other person and a sense that this is now more difficult; difficulties with communication; carers missing activities they used to be able to do with the person with dementia; and a sense that carers bear the brunt of the frustrations of the person they care for.

For carers, the ability to share activities with the person they care for is important. This can include special events such as holidays and day trips, but also everyday activities such as gardening, cooking or visiting the library. Visiting a library potentially offers carers a chance to share an activity that both the person with dementia and their carer enjoy, such as reading groups or arts activities. Libraries also offer carers time to follow their own interests, for example by choosing books or other resources that appeal to them personally. It is therefore important that carers feel welcome in the library and are aware that the staff understand appropriate ways of supporting people with dementia. For example, this might mean being confident that staff will support them and help to smooth over any misunderstandings with other customers if the person with dementia says or does something that would normally be considered inappropriate in that setting.

Support for library staff affected by dementia

Of course, libraries need to focus on the needs of customers; but it is important to remember that dementia will also affect members of library staff in a variety of ways – and with the projected growth in dementia cases over the coming decades, the number of staff affected is likely to increase.

Around the world, individual countries will have specific legislation that outlines the ways in which people with dementia and those who care for them should be supported in the workplace. For instance, in the UK, under the Equality Act 2010, employers are required to make reasonable adjustments for people with disabilities, including people with dementia, to ensure they are not disadvantaged at work. This section does not discuss such legal requirements in detail as these will vary in different territories, but instead outlines some of the common practical approaches taken by employers.

Support for staff with dementia

Studies have shown that, when well supported, many people with dementia can continue working, which for some can mean they are able to retain skills and feel they are continuing to contribute economically and socially to society (Ritchie et al., 2017). However, many people with dementia stop working – sometimes through choice, but often because the level of support that will enable them to continue in their jobs is not available. In the UK, for example, only 18% of people diagnosed with dementia under the age of 65 continue to work after their diagnosis (Alzheimer's Society, 2015b).

Appropriate support for a person with dementia in the workplace depends on the type of employment, the symptoms the person currently experiences and the resources available. It is therefore important to take a person-centred approach to supporting continued employment. For example, someone who is primarily experiencing memory problems will require different types of support from someone experiencing visuospatial issues, and someone working in a customer service role will need different adjustments to someone whose primary role is in conservation and collection care.

Physical changes to the workplace may help, for example moving the person's desk to a quieter area; installing soundproofing or visual barriers to minimise distractions; having clear signage to enable the person to find their way around the building; adopting a clear labelling system to help the person organise their work; or designing dementia-friendly meeting spaces. The employer may also need to provide extra aids or support, such as quality checking systems, written instructions or the use of memory cues such as team calendars, diaries and mobile phone alerts. Support from a 'buddy', or some form of mentoring or counselling support, is another way in which an employer can provide support for an employee with dementia.

Sometimes a change in job description – for example, a reduction in the number of tasks, responsibilities or hours worked – may be appropriate. However, if changes to working hours or level of responsibility are being considered, there may be financial implications for the employee that need to be considered too. In addition, if the employee is finding it more difficult to learn new things, then moving to another job – even what might be considered a less challenging one – could be counterproductive. Changes to working patterns, such as adjusted start and finish times or homeworking options, may be helpful in some cases, for example if someone's symptoms tend to be worse in the mornings or evenings.

It is not just day-to-day work tasks where adjustments need to be made. It is also important that people with dementia can access training opportunities. Some examples of possible adjustments include tailoring training techniques to suit individual needs; ensuring trainers are flexible and able to accommodate the person's needs; ensuring that venues, resources and visual aids are accessible; allowing additional time for activities; or modifying instructions and handouts.

Whatever workplace adjustments are made, it is important to hold regular meetings to ensure that these have been implemented effectively and are still meeting the individual's needs, as well as making the staff member aware of the support available from trade unions, staff associations, occupational health, counselling services, disability support networks and other support services.

Even when all possible adjustments have been made or discussed, the person with dementia may feel that they do not want to continue at work. As part of the information provided to help the employee make this transition, such as guidance on access to advice on benefits and pensions, it may be appropriate to explore opportunities for volunteering within the library service that fit with the person's skill set. Some people may find it enjoyable and therapeutic to return to aspects of work, but on a more informal basis, and maintain contact with their colleagues in a familiar environment.

Support for staff caring for someone with dementia

In most library services, there will likely be members of staff who are caring for a family member with dementia. In the UK, for example, half of all carers (3.25 million people) juggle paid work alongside caring. Whilst this figure includes all carers, research has shown full-time working carers are most likely to be caring for someone with dementia (Carers UK/EfC, 2014).

Research by Carers UK investigated the impact of caring for someone with dementia on people's capacity to work. Just over half of respondents (53%) said that their work had been negatively affected due to their caring responsibilities (through tiredness, anxiety, stress, etc.). Almost 1 in 4 said that they had changed their working pattern; 1 in 5 had reduced their working hours; and 1 in 10 had taken a less qualified/less senior role to fit around their caring responsibilities. Only 7% of carers reported that caring had not had an impact on their capacity to work (Carers UK/EfC, 2014).

Common types of support offered to carers include flexible working arrangements and flexible/special leave (paid and/or unpaid) to allow them to take time off when they need to. Other types of help can include signposting employees to other sources of support they may be able to access; practical help to support the employee's own health and wellbeing; awareness raising events to make other staff more aware of the types of issues colleagues may be facing; remote working; and a workplace carers' network. However, there is clearly still much to be done to improve – and to publicise – workplace support for carers. The Carers UK research described above found that 18% of carers said there was no specific support provided at their workplace and a further 13% did not know whether there was support available (Carers UK/EfC, 2014).

Support for volunteers

Whilst some forms of support, such as leave arrangements, are only applicable to paid staff, it is important to remember that many libraries will also have volunteers who are caring for someone with dementia. For some people in a caring role, volunteering is important in providing them with an opportunity to explore their own interests and have a short respite from caring responsibilities. If the library (or in some cases its parent organisation) provides support such as carers' networks or signposting to organisations that can offer help, it may be appropriate to extend this to volunteers too. In addition, as Charlotte Sumner, Team Leader at Paignton Library in the UK describes, simply making sure there is someone who is able and willing to listen to volunteers (or indeed other staff members) can be an important form of support:

> It's very difficult, because there's not much you can proactively do apart from be there to listen to someone sometimes. Most weeks when the volunteers are in, it's the same sort of conversations you have, because they need to get it off their chest and just have someone to talk to really . . . I think it's just being a person to talk to.
>
> (C. Sumner, conversation with author, 8 December 2021)

Support for staff working alongside someone with dementia

Research has highlighted the impact that having a colleague diagnosed with dementia can have on co-workers (Ritchie et al., 2017). As well as experiencing increased workloads, there can be an emotional impact on colleagues who work with a person with dementia. As Charlotte Sumner's comment above indicates, staff may often need to provide emotional support for people with dementia or for carers in their workplace. Supporting a colleague with dementia can be stressful, especially in the pre-diagnosis stages when problems are emerging, and neither the person themselves nor those around them are certain what is causing the changes. This can lead to conflicts within the workplace. Later, once someone has a diagnosis, staff may experience feelings of guilt over not recognising the earlier signs of dementia in their colleague.

Given the lack of understanding of dementia across society as a whole and the often negative portrayals of the condition (described in the Introduction), it is not surprising that colleagues may struggle to understand how best to interact with and support a person with dementia in the workplace. Holding an awareness session on dementia can be helpful, perhaps involving the person with dementia directly in delivering this if it is something they feel comfortable with. Further training options to help staff better support both customers and colleagues are outlined below.

Training opportunities

This chapter has provided an overview of some of the ways in which library staff can provide support for people with dementia and their carers. However, to do this effectively, staff need opportunities to develop a better understanding of the needs of people affected by dementia. This final section briefly outlines some of the training opportunities available that may be useful for library staff, as well as volunteers – and indeed have already been taken up by staff in many library services. Of course, training courses produced in one country or region may contain information specific to that territory. However, the general principles in the training outlined below will be applicable to library staff elsewhere too.

Dementia Friends

Dementia Friends was developed by the UK Alzheimer's Society (2017b). It is open to anyone and helps people to understand more about dementia and the small, everyday ways in which they can help to make their community more dementia friendly. Becoming a Dementia Friend involves attending an information session (face-to-face or online) to learn about what it is like to live with dementia and then turning that understanding into practical actions that could help someone living in their community. Several local councils in the UK have actively supported the roll out of Dementia Friends by promoting the training amongst council staff (including library staff) and officials. Dementia Friends Champions are volunteers trained by the Alzheimer's Society to deliver Dementia Friends sessions in their workplaces and communities.

Dementia awareness e-learning course

The UK Social Care Institute of Excellence has produced a free e-learning course on dementia awareness (SCIE, 2019). This is primarily designed for care staff, but much of the material is also relevant to library staff who want more in-depth information than is provided through Dementia Friends training. Learning outcomes from the course include: understanding the importance of recognising what is important to people; how dementia affects the person, their family and wider society; how to communicate effectively and compassionately with individuals who have dementia; and how to respond effectively to people with dementia who have different communication needs.

Locally organised training: Wisconsin Libraries

Whilst some training opportunities have been developed by national organisations, there may also be opportunities to provide training for library staff by drawing on local networks and partnerships. An example is the Dementia Friendly (Purple Angel) Training in Wisconsin in the United States. Library staff within many Wisconsin communities have received training as part of dementia-friendly community initiatives. The training may be completed by a Dementia Care Specialist or staff members from the local Aging and Disability Resource Center (ADRC), Alzheimer's Association chapter or the Alzheimer's and Dementia Alliance of Wisconsin office. The training typically includes information on the signs and symptoms of dementia, effective communication strategies for people with memory loss and how to create a safe and welcoming environment for people with cognitive issues and their care partners. Once the library has received the dementia-friendly designation, most provide ongoing training to existing staff and volunteers, as well as to new team members (Wisconsin Alzheimer's Institute, 2017).

Dementia-Friendly Canada online education

Whilst there are now training opportunities similar to those described above available for library staff to access in many countries and regions, most of the current training is generic and there are few examples of training specifically tailored to the needs of library staff. However, as part of the Dementia-Friendly Canada project, online education in Building Dementia-Friendly Communities has been created specifically for the 'Recreation and Library' sector (as well as training for staff in 'Restaurant and Retail' and 'Public Transportation'). This national project is led by the Alzheimer Society of Canada, with contributions from provincial Alzheimer Societies. It builds on previous work such as the Dementia Friendly Toolkit for Libraries (Alzheimer Society of Saskatchewan, 2019) described above. The course provides a foundational knowledge of dementia and outlines the considerations that organisations can include in their social and physical environments to better support and include people living with dementia (Alzheimer Society of Canada, 2022).

Heather Cowie, National Project Manager for Dementia-Friendly Canada describes the development of the course, and why she feels it is important to have library-specific training materials:

> My colleagues in each province had conversations with people living with dementia and care partners about what services they access in their communities that they'd like to feel more supported in. Three key sectors emerged: public transportation; retail and restaurant; and recreation and library. We created education modules by pulling from existing resources and from holding focus groups with people in these industries. In these, we learnt that people wanted their education to be modular and self-paced. After piloting the course, we found these participants showed significant increase in their knowledge and confidence when interacting with people affected by dementia.
>
> My dream is to have everyone educated, which is part of the reason we created the course to be online and easily accessible – that way we can reach as many people as possible. After they have the initial knowledge, we hope they are inspired to learn more. While the education modules in the course have the same core content, they have very specific examples for the activities of each sector – this is because people want to ensure they can see themselves in those situations.
>
> Obviously, we want to change the world, but we're realistic. In our physical environment module, for instance, we were really cognisant that you can't just tear down your library and rebuild it from scratch to be dementia friendly. But there are simple and affordable things you can change: you can work on your signage to be clear and legible and you make sure the step strips are clear and easy to see. Also, you can work on your communication, so that if you recognise

someone's having difficulties, you could go over and help. So what Alzheimer Societies really promote is bettering your communication, knowing when you can help and knowing when you should refer back to us to learn a little bit more.
(Heather Cowie, e-mail to author, 9 June 2022)

Conclusions

This chapter has focused on how libraries as organisations can play an important role in the creation of dementia-friendly communities, but also how individual staff can contribute to making sure that people with dementia and their carers feel welcome and included in the library. The importance of library staff having some level of understanding of dementia – and a positive attitude towards people with dementia – cannot be underestimated. The next three chapters look in greater detail at library design and environment; reading activities; and health, social and arts activities. However, if the fundamental building block of staff knowledge is not in place, much of the good achieved through the dementia-friendly design of spaces or activities can be lost. My experiences of researching case studies for this book highlighted the importance of staff knowledge, especially for those in front line roles, and I reflect further on this in the following chapters. I would agree with the comments made by Heather Cowie from Dementia-Friendly Canada: staff need to see how dementia-friendly principles apply to their own workplace to truly understand them. Hopefully, in the future, there will be more training and support that does just that.

3
Library Design and Environment

> For all the things we cannot change in the room, the most important thing we learned was the importance of greater awareness amongst staff.
> (Mari Gudim Torp, Deichman Oppsal Library, Norway, in e-mail to author)

This chapter explores the ways in which library spaces and environments can be organised with people with dementia in mind. Aspects of design discussed include signage, colour schemes, layout, furnishing and lighting. A series of case studies illustrate how these principles have been put into practice in libraries. Some of the examples discussed are the result of large-scale building or refurbishment projects. Whilst not all libraries are in a position to make such dramatic changes to their building structure, many of the ideas described are small changes that can be introduced, often at minimal cost, in existing library environments. As the quote above from Mari Gudim Torp at Deichman Oppsal Library in Norway emphasises, creating a dementia-friendly library is not purely a task for architects and designers. These professionals can do a great deal to put the initial building blocks in place, but in the longer term, it is down to library staff and managers to ensure that library environments remain dementia friendly on a day-to-day basis.

Of course, a library should feel friendly and welcoming to everyone. However, this can be particularly important to people with dementia. It is crucial to remember that, although an accessible building is helpful, people with dementia say that it is the people in the building who make all the difference. Friendly, welcoming staff can override many design problems (DEEP, 2013).

There is detailed guidance available relating to the design of dementia-friendly public spaces. In the UK, for instance, the Dementia Services Development Centre (DSDC) at the University of Stirling has produced a set of standards for dementia-friendly design and runs a building accreditation scheme. Whilst these standards are not written specifically with libraries in mind, much of the following advice, as summarised by the UK Dementia Action Alliance (DAA, n.d.), is likely to be applicable to library buildings.

1. A person with dementia in the building will feel calm and relaxed.
2. The building is familiar: consideration has been given to age- and culturally-appropriate design.
3. The layout of the building is easy to understand.
4. There are high levels of visibility. This means that, as far as possible, people can see where they need to go since they may be unable to remember, or work out the layout.
5. There is plenty of light – both natural and artificial.
6. Confusing patterns in surfaces, fabrics and floor coverings, such as specks, sparkle or stripes, have been avoided.
7. The floor is a consistent colour without contrasting threshold strips.
8. Surfaces are not shiny or reflective as these can be confusing and can make floors look slippery or wet.
9. Dead-end corridors have been avoided. These cause frustration.
10. The building is quiet: overstimulation from noise can be distressing for people with dementia. Noise can be reduced in numerous ways, including with sound-absorbing materials/panels.
11. There is somewhere quiet to go, away from the main activity area.
12. All toilet doors are the same: easy to see and have the same clear sign.
13. There is good colour/tonal contrast in the toilets, making it easy to identify handrails, toilet seat, controls, etc. The soap dispenser and taps are easy to see and understand how to operate.
14. Different rooms (or sections of the library) that have different functions have plenty of cues as to the purpose of the room (or section). Colour/tonal contrast is used to make things clear.
15. There is good directional signage. Signage combines words and a clear picture, contrasts with the background and is mounted no more than 1.2 metres from the floor.

This guidance gives a good overview, but it is worth looking at some key aspects of dementia-friendly design in more detail and considering how these might apply to a library building. Some of the considerations discussed below are principles of good library design in general or aspects of inclusive design that libraries need to consider in order to meet the needs of disabled people and other users. However, it is worth recapping these here in more detail as they are likely to be especially important for people with dementia using the library building.

Finding the library

The first challenge for someone with dementia can be simply finding the library. A dementia-friendly library needs to be easy to locate and identify. Of course, this is easier to achieve in some cases than others; the historical location of a library may mean it is not always in the most prominent location. If the library is located off the main street, for example, it is important to explore what signage is possible to direct people who may not know (or remember) exactly where to go. Including an image of each branch library on the library service website and in publicity leaflets is a simple measure that can be helpful as potential customers then know what the library building looks like before they visit.

When someone does see the building, its purpose – the fact that it is a library – should be obvious. However, this can be more problematic than it might at first seem, especially with co-located services or rebranded libraries. Buildings labelled 'Idea Store', 'Lifestyle Centre', 'One Stop Shop' and so forth may well not be obvious as a library to someone with dementia – and potentially other customers too.

Once someone has found the library, it needs to be easy to get into the building: the entrance should be clearly visible and obviously indicated as an entrance. Lighting at entrances should be bright and include natural light when possible – but avoid pools of bright light and deep shadows, which can be confusing. Think about key points where people are likely to need signage, for example in the car park to show how to get into the building or to the library itself if this is in a multi-function building. In larger buildings in particular, it is helpful to have a reception area near the entrance with a member of staff to greet people and direct them.

Step-free access is important, with a ramp or lift if necessary. If this is not available at the main entrance, make sure the step-free access point is clearly signed. Revolving doors may also cause difficulties.

Getting around the library

Once they are inside the library, there are a number of ways in which it can be made easier for someone with dementia to find their way around. This includes signage and layout, but also aspects such as wall colour, floor coverings, lighting and furnishings.

Signage and layout

Signage is important to help people with dementia find their way around the library as they may not remember the layout even if they have been visiting for several years. Signs should be easy to read in clear, bold text and where appropriate include an understandable picture that indicates the meaning of the sign in an unambiguous way in addition to the words. Matt surfaces are generally easier to read as they avoid glare, so avoid signs made of reflective materials. There should be a good contrast between the text and the background colour of the sign. There should also be a clear contrast between the sign and the surface it is attached to, so the sign stands out. Ideally, signs should be fixed to the doors they refer to, rather than on the wall next to them, and be easily visible at eye level – not too high or too low.

If the library has signage hanging from the ceiling, consider adding additional navigational aids on shelving or walls. Whilst you may not always be able to control or change the design of signage, there are ways to improve the signage you already have. For example, make sure that there is space around signs and that walls are not cluttered with posters and notices. Signs for toilets and exits are particularly important. In enclosed areas, such as toilets, remember to include signs showing how to get back to the main library as someone may have forgotten where they came in.

As well as explicit signage, having 'landmarks' at key places in the library can be helpful, for example a large artwork at the entrance/exit. This can help people to 'get their bearings', and creates a familiar landscape for someone with dementia to move around in the space, minimising anxiety they may feel through being in an unfamiliar location. In addition, a large calendar with the day, date and month, plus a clock with large numbers (Arabic rather than Roman numerals) and ideally an indication of the time of day (i.e. morning or afternoon) can help a person with dementia to orientate themselves in the library.

In general, try to keep the layout of the library as open as possible so people can see where they need to go – lower shelving heights can make this easier. It is advisable to avoid having corridors or passages that come to dead ends, although obviously this is easier in some buildings than others. Also, avoid changing the layout of the library frequently. Occasionally you may need to rearrange the layout of course, so be aware that people with dementia are likely to need additional support to navigate the new space and staff should look out for anyone who may need help.

As mentioned above, helpful staff can be crucial in overcoming any issues around the building design or layout that are difficult to overcome through simple adjustments. Unlike services such as banks and public transport, library staff do not usually wear uniforms, so name tags with writing in a contrasting colour font and large letters can help customers to identify staff members if they want to ask for help.

Walls and other surfaces

As described above, making sure the library is as open as possible is important. Being able to see between different areas can also assist orientation. However, glazed doors can cause confusion and, potentially, accidents. Glazing should therefore be highlighted by the use of 'manifestations' (clearly visible patterns on glass) and any fixed glazed screens should be distinguished from glass doors or openings. It is important to be aware that reflective surfaces can cause confusing reflections, exacerbate visual-perceptual difficulties and potentially cause distress for some people with dementia. It is therefore best to avoid mirrors if possible, but in particular avoid placing them where they are most likely to cause confusion, for example at the end of a hallway or opposite a door.

Doors that blend into the wall can be difficult to see, so publicly accessible doors or entrance frames should be painted in a contrasting colour to walls. However, non-accessible doors (for example, to staff-only areas) can be painted to blend in with walls so people are not encouraged to go through them.

Flooring

To help people with dementia to orientate themselves, the floor should be a different colour to the walls of a room. Within the floor design itself, avoid too much contrast, bold patterns and changes in tone. Stripes can look like steps and flecked flooring can look like something has been dropped onto the floor. As with other surfaces, highly shiny floors are best avoided. Take care with mats as these can be trip hazards – for people with or without dementia. Furthermore, for some people with dementia, dark mats can appear as holes in the ground and blue mats can look like pools of water.

Joins between flooring in adjacent areas that you want library customers to be able to easily cross between should not be too obvious. Likewise, try to avoid any flooring repairs appearing too noticeable as this could cause confusion and hesitation. On some occasions, however, you will want to indicate where people need to be aware of a change in the flooring. Steps are an obvious example; there should be a contrast between treads and risers so that people can clearly see where to put their feet; for example, marking the edges of dark coloured steps with yellow strips.

Furnishings

Plain fabrics or subtle patterns are the saftest choice for furnishings; bold or complex patterns can lead to confusion as, to someone with dementia, the patterns may appear to move. Textures that are attractive to the touch can be soothing and reassuring. There are various 'fiddle' products available for people with dementia, such as sensory cushions or blankets made of contrasting fabrics that people can explore as a way to focus on an activity or simply to relax.

While it is not necessary to try to reproduce the past – people with dementia will have memories from a number of different eras in any event – do ensure that the furnishings look like their intended purpose. For example, modern designs of some chairs and benches may mean they are not instantly recognisable to everyone as something you are expected to sit on.

When considering the colour scheme of the library, be aware that people with dementia (and older people in general) tend to lose colour vision from the blue end of the spectrum first. The use of warmer, brighter colours in furnishings and other décor across the library can therefore help to make things more visible. In particular, it may be difficult for people to differentiate shades of blue and green, so avoid using these colours to signify different features or areas of the library that people need to distinguish from each other.

Lighting

Of course, as many customers are going to read in the library, lighting needs to be good, but again this is something that is particularly important for people with dementia. Daylight should be made use of wherever possible. Artificial lighting is also likely to be needed, but this should be evenly spread to avoid confusing shadows or patterns forming on the floor. In addition, try to avoid glare or flickering lights.

If customers need to be able to control lights themselves (for example, in toilets), switch plate covers in a contrasting colour can improve the visibility of light switches. Motion sensor lights can be useful as customers do not have to find a light switch, but make sure these are set correctly. If the light switches off completely (rather than dimming to a low level) when it is not in use, this can lead to confusion and possibly panic if the lights turn off whilst someone is using the toilet.

Lifts

The flooring in lifts should be the same tone as the floor outside and the threshold should also be a similar tone to both floor surfaces. Ideally, reflective or shiny surfaces should be avoided for the walls of the lift. If a mirror is necessary for wheelchair users, an angled one at a high level can be used. The lift should have a handrail. Buttons in the lift should be big, clear and easy to press, and ideally there should be an announcement system to announce arrival at different floors.

Case studies of dementia-friendly library design

So far, this chapter has outlined some general principles of library design that can help to make the environment more dementia friendly. The cases studies below describe how these principles have been put into practice in libraries. Even though some of these describe major refurbishments or building projects, they all include examples of basic ideas that would be possible in most libraries without the need for major investment.

Warrington (Livewire) Libraries, UK

Public libraries in Warrington in the northwest of England are run by Livewire, a community interest company (CIC) that looks after leisure, library and lifestyle services. Several libraries in the locality have been designed, or refurbished, to make them more dementia friendly.

Great Sankey Neighbourhood Hub

Great Sankey Neighbourhood Hub in Warrington, a new build that opened in 2018, aims to provide integrated cultural, leisure and health provision to promote wellness and wellbeing. The building, located in a suburb close to Warrington town centre, comprises sports facilities, a spa and meeting rooms, as well as a public library. The brief for this complex project was developed in consultation with stakeholders including LiveWire, the Borough Council, Sport England, Warrington Disability Partnership, Warrington Clinical Commissioning Group (National Health Service (NHS) bodies responsible for the planning and commissioning of health care services for their local area), Warrington Dementia Action Alliance and Culture Warrington, which manages cultural venues in the town. The team worked closely with academic experts from the University of Stirling to meet the criteria for their DSDC Gold Award, which was achieved in 2019. Full accreditation had not been attempted for a multi-use public building before and the team worked with the University and Walker Simpson Architects (WSA) to adapt and develop design principles that were previously only in existence for specialist facilities such as care homes and hospitals. Attention was paid to various aspects of the design, including colour contrasts; levels of natural and artificial lighting; acoustics; furniture and fittings; and signage.

A ten-point plan was compiled by LiveWire and WSA highlighting design features that make Great Sankey Neighbourhood Hub a dementia-friendly building:

1. A clear and legible building layout to assist orientation.
2. Entrance and exits are clearly signposted to assist wayfinding.
3. Recognisable furniture and fittings, for example seating and analogue clocks, for familiarity, comfort and timekeeping.
4. Seating with backrests and armrests is available throughout the building, with ergonomic design principles for user comfort and frequent opportunities for sitting.
5. High contrasts between floors, walls, doors and objects. Large-scale, contrasting patterns are avoided.
6. Clear signage with upper- and lower-case letters and graphic symbols positioned at appropriate heights. Public signage is larger and more visible than ancillary room signage.
7. Public doors are emphasised whereas ancillary doors are 'hidden' to avoid visual 'clutter' for users and to assist wayfinding.
8. Toilet facilities are directly available along main circulation routes, and doors have a signature colour strip.
9. Good daylighting levels with views to the outside to help orientation.
10. Memory box display cabinets and large reminiscence images are curated with assistance from Culture Warrington to promote a feeling of familiarity and comfort. (Mark Rathbone, e-mail to author, 25 November 2021)

LiveWire launched a dementia-friendly activity programme that includes specifically designed group exercise classes, quiet hours in the gym and dementia-friendly swimming times. Staff have received special training in order to raise awareness of dementia and the impact it can have on people and on their family and friends.

The building includes a small library in the concourse area of the building, immediately accessible from the entrance lobby. This has been designed to provide both books and a digital offer, with a children's library at the centre of the space. However, the library service in the Hub is not confined to a single location but is dispersed throughout the building: there are book carousels and shelves in different zones with some themed areas such as 'Dementia and Health' and 'Fitness and Activity'.

Locating a library within a multi-function facility is inevitably challenging (McNicol, 2008) and particularly so if the space is also intended to be dementia friendly. Whilst the building at Great Sankey Neighbourhood Hub has been designed to include many dementia-friendly features, it also highlights the need to be aware of library-specific considerations. For instance, features that may be well-suited to one facility, such as music and PA announcements usual in a gym, can be less conducive to the use of library resources. The lack of specialist library staff can also be challenging. Not always having dedicated staff available to support customers and to manage the collection and the library space on a day-to-day basis may make the library more difficult to use for some people, especially in the absence of a great deal of library-specific signage, such as shelf labels or instructions on how to borrow books located in different areas of the building.

Stockton Heath Library
Following the development of Great Sankey, LiveWire has been keen to introduce aspects of dementia-friendly design into other local libraries too. Nearby Stockton Heath Library reopened in September 2019 following a refurbishment. This case study illustrates the important role of library staff in maintaining a dementia-friendly design to ensure it remains as accessible as possible in the long term, after the designers have left.

Mark Rathbone, Project Advisor at LiveWire, describes the process of refurbishing Stockton Heath Library and provides an example of the added contribution staff can bring:

> We were limited by the existing building structure and a tight budget of course. However, we have still applied as many of the key features of dementia-friendly design as possible including clear layout, clearer signage, avoiding contrasting patterns, improved daylighting levels and softer lighting and a few 'homely' touches by the staff, including some beautiful flower displays!
>
> A lot of this is common-sense design, but it's a fantastic opportunity to re-think our buildings in the same way that improved accessibility requirements or health and safety regulations have done in the past. A good example of this is signage and wayfinding, ensuring clear routes and clear lines of sight and avoiding sharp colour contrasts, particularly on the flooring. Sudden changes in colour or style can be seen as a barrier, or a step or a hole by someone with dementia, but so many libraries still retain their 1970s/1980s colour schemes or 'chequer board' carpet tile designs which are not fit for that purpose.
>
> (Mark Rathbone, e-mail to author, 25 November 2021)

Stockton Heath Library has clear signage, with labels on all shelves to indicate the different sections of stock and a large sign on the wall that can be seen from around the library to show the location of the self-service issue machine. There are also clear signs on doors, with those leading to staff areas painted in a similar colour to walls, whilst the customer toilet door is painted to stand out. Noticeboards are well-organised and clearly labelled (for example, 'What's On', 'Children's Information'). There is a quiet room off the main library, as well as a children's library, which has walls painted in a contrasting colour to the adult areas. There is also a pleasant seating area with plenty of chairs with high seats and armrests that make it easier for someone to stand up. As Mark commented above, the part played by staff in keeping the space dementia friendly is evident at Stockton Heath Library; for example, in making sure the entrance is kept clear and the library tidy and free of clutter that could be confusing or even a trip hazard.

Kirklees Libraries, UK

In Kirklees, a district in the north of England, the decision to develop dementia-friendly public libraries is also part of a broader local authority initiative. Kirklees Council has worked with the University of Stirling to produce a Dementia-Friendly Design Tool (DSDC, 2021). The Tool is a collection of guidance that supports dementia-friendly design, layout and furnishing in various types of buildings and spaces. It helps provide practical solutions to ensure places and spaces around Kirklees are inclusive for people living with dementia. This Tool can be used by anyone, from homeowners wishing to make simple domestic changes to business owners, service providers and construction professionals. To encourage different types of organisations and businesses to make changes, there is guidance specifically for different building typologies, including outdoor environments; eating, drinking and socialising; activity and leisure; and public buildings.

In addition to general guidance on topics such as patterns and colour, light levels, and signage and wayfinding, the Tool has a section on library-specific guidance as part of the activity and leisure section. Advice includes:

- introducing light tones in the colour scheme and décor to enable light reflection off more surfaces
- incorporating artwork of cultural significance or by local artists
- lowering bookshelf heights to enable people to see all books on offer and provide sight lines over the top of cases to assist wayfinding
- allowing ample space for a wheelchair to manoeuvre without obstacles. (DSDC, 2021)

This guidance has informed the development of dementia-friendly libraries in Kirklees, including Almondbury Library.

Almondbury Library

In 2019 Almondbury Library moved to a new Community Hub where local residents can access a range of services under one roof, including support for children and families; help and advice; activities for older people; community events; and library services. Located just outside Huddersfield town centre, it was the first dementia-friendly library in the district. The library is located off the main road in a quiet corner of the village and there is a care home close by.

The welcome desk is visible from the library entrance and there is a large clock above showing the day and date, as well as the time. Although it is a relatively small space, the bookshelves at Almondbury Library are arranged so that there are no dead ends. The broad genre of books (for example, fiction, non-fiction) is indicated by non-reflective shelf-top signs with large, clear lettering. There is a small dementia collection near the entrance with books and information about local dementia support services. The majority of flyers displayed on noticeboards are not laminated, making them easier to read. There are plenty of chairs with arms, including dining-style chairs around a table and a more relaxed seating area, but still with fairly high seats that are easier to stand up from. The chairs and seat cushions are made from plain fabrics in vivid colours that contrast with the library carpet and walls.

Sandal Library, Wakefield, UK

Sandal Library is a small branch library in a residential area just outside Wakefield town centre in northern England. The library received a major refurbishment in 2015, making it one of the first UK libraries designed to be fully dementia friendly. The interior was redesigned, in partnership with the Alzheimer's Society, to help people living with dementia to feel comfortable, supported and more independent.

There is large, clear signage on the front of the library building and an accessible entrance with a ramp and rails. Inside, the décor uses flat colours rather than patterns. There are grey skirting boards and door frames to create well-defined entrances and exits against magnolia walls. There is plain carpeting and no contrast-coloured mats that can look like holes in the ground. Reflective surfaces are minimised: the designers did not install mirrors; avoided using chrome legs on tables and chairs; and applied a specially designed decal to cover the glazed sliding entrance/exit doors.

The furniture is conventional in style, with wood finishes to provide a warmer, more traditional feel. The designers opted for deep red for chairs, signage and other furnishings. There are symbols to accompany text signs, for example to indicate where different genres of books can be found. A large display screen shows the day, date and time in both analogue and digital formats.

Sandal Library has a reminiscence area located off the main library in an area that has good natural light, with a magic table (see Chapter 6) and reminiscence displays and resources. This area is decorated with artwork created by local artists and members of the library's Active Minds group, which holds regular events with quizzes, games, crafts, reminiscence and conversation. There is also access to a community garden at the rear of the library.

The library generated a 73% surge in visits in the year after it opened; many of those were new users and many were attracted specifically by the dementia-friendly environment (Shared Intelligence, 2017). Since the refurbishment at Sandal, elements of the dementia-friendly design have been adopted in other branch libraries in Wakefield, including clear signage; traditional-style furnishings in plain fabric; clearly defined entrances, exits and wall edges; reminiscence displays; and large clocks displaying the day and time (Clarke, 2022).

Belper Library, Derbyshire, UK

Belper is located within the Derwent Valley Mills UNESCO World Heritage Site in Derbyshire. The area was designated by UNESCO in 2001 because it was one of the first modern industrial settlements constructed as part of the introduction of the factory system in the 18th century (Derwent Valley Mills, n.d.). Belper Library is located in a formerly derelict chocolate factory, which was part-refurbished and part-rebuilt to house a public library, as well as a café and the Ada Belfield Centre, a local authority-owned care home. The existing historical facades of the factory were retained, refurbished and incorporated into the new building design. The library, which opened in 2020, showcases much of the original architecture, potentially stimulating memories for older people who remember the building as a working factory.

There is a public café at the entrance to the building. The care home and library, which are located in separate wings, are clearly signed. The library has good natural light and pleasant seating areas – both in the library itself and in a sunny alcove just outside – with traditional-style seating with arms to make it easier for people who are less mobile to stand up. There are separate children's and teenage areas, as well as a local studies section located off the main library. There is large, clear signage on the bookshelves and paintings by a local art group are displayed around the library. The majority of the shelving is curved, which helps to maintain sight lines to the entrance/exit as you browse the shelves. There are well-organised noticeboards near the entrance with information about library services as well as local events and activities.

The care home located on the same site has a library ticket for their residents. Library staff select books for residents and some residents visit the library themselves. COVID-19 restrictions in care homes have limited activities since the library opened, but staff hope to develop activities in the library for care home residents in the future (S. Royle, e-mail to author, 26 May 2022).

Deichman Oppsal Library, Oslo, Norway

Whilst the case studies described so far show how dementia-friendly design has been incorporated as part of library new builds or refurbishments, Deichman Oppsal Library in Oslo undertook a project to explore ways to make an existing public library more dementia friendly. Whilst there are elements of the case studies discussed so far that can be incorporated within existing libraries, the approach taken by Deichman Oppsal is one that is likely to be especially relevant to many library services. It demonstrates that it may not be necessary to wait until there is funding available for a major refurbishment before making adjustments to make a library more dementia-friendly; there is much that can be achieved with a smaller level of investment and drawing on local community expertise.

Deichman Oppsal undertook a pilot project in 2018 to better understand how libraries can meet the needs of older people and people with dementia. The project undertook extensive consultation with older people, people with dementia, library staff and professionals with dementia-friendliness competence to identify measures that could help make the venue age- and dementia-friendly. Some key areas identified were clear physical surroundings; colours and contrasts; markings and signage; sight and lighting; and hearing and noise. Some of the adjustments made to the library as a result included:

- doors to rooms with non-public functions (for example, staff areas) painted in the same colour as the wall to blend in
- toilet doors painted in a contrasting colour to the walls and new signs added with a symbol and large-font text
- step edges marked with tape and furniture placed so that the step edges are more visible
- new bookshelf signs to make it easier to find books
- signage in a contrasting colour to the walls and in large sentence-case font with symbols to indicate important features such as the information desk
- spot lighting installed over reading areas, sofa seating groups and the loan machine, and positioned to avoid reflections or glare
- sound-absorbing panels mounted in the ceiling to reduce loud noises
- signposts to the information desk and a bell with a sign added to make it easier to call for help
- events especially for people with dementia
- staff available to support people during events and provide details such as the length of activities, refreshment arrangements and location of toilets
- a 'short and sweet' shelf with easy-to-read books, short texts and short stories
- a 'listening station' for audio books, added in collaboration with the Norwegian Audio and Braille Library
- greater awareness amongst staff; for example, supporting people who are unable to use the self-service loan machine or have forgotten their PIN
- issuing staff with lanyards so they are more visible to customers whilst walking around the library.

As this was a pilot project, it was not possible to achieve everything the library wanted to. In the future, Deichman Oppsal hopes to incorporate further dementia-friendly features such as more suitable furniture with higher seats and armrests that are easier to get up from, as well as accessories such as cushions and tablecloths that are dementia friendly in terms of colours and contrasts used (M. Gudim Torp, e-mail to author, 21 January 2021)

Sensory spaces

In addition to considering ways to make the library building as a whole dementia friendly, some libraries have added specific facilities such as sensory spaces or immersive experience rooms designed for people with dementia, as well as for those with other conditions such as autism, learning disabilities or anxiety. Sensory therapy, sometimes called Snoezelen therapy, has been used for a number of years for people with dementia. It aims to stimulate the senses through features such as lighting effects; tactile surfaces; meditative music or sounds; and aromatherapy oils (Sánchez et al., 2013). Sensory rooms are often located in care homes, but having these types of facilities located within libraries potentially opens up this therapy to people with dementia living in the community.

In recent years several libraries have developed sensory rooms, but in most cases these appear to be primarily targeted towards children with autism or learning disabilities, and their parents. The potential of sensory rooms to provide a quiet, calm and soothing space, or to offer sensory stimulation, for people with dementia seems to be underexploited at present. Informal conversations I had whilst researching this book suggest that there is, perhaps, a need for greater training and awareness-raising for library staff to ensure they are aware that, where a sensory room is available, it can cater for different needs depending on the ways in which the resources are configured and used.

Immersive experience room, Stockton-on-Tees Libraries and Archives, UK

A sensory facility that has been used effectively by people with dementia is the Imagination Station at Thornaby Central Library in Stockton-on-Tees in the UK, which opened in 2018. This space provides sensory and immersive experiences for older people; people living with dementia, autism, sensory or learning disabilities; or those who simply need a quiet space. Interestingly, in the context of dementia provision, the room can be used to project historical or reminiscence images, as well as images and sounds intended to promote relaxation. Karen Morris, Health and Wellbeing Librarian at Stockton-on-Tees Borough Council, describes one way in which this facility can be used by people with dementia. Whilst not having a separate room to hold their dementia café could be challenging, library staff are able to make use of the Imagination Station as somewhere people can go to relax if they are feeling overwhelmed.

> We have our dementia café, which is an open forum and there are members of the public coming in and out all the time. We don't have a separate room; we run it in the middle of the library. There are so many things to take into consideration when you're running something with people with dementia: you've got to think of noise; you've got to think how much there is going on around; whether they're going to be overstimulated; whether they feel uncomfortable. But we have our immersive experience room called an Imagination Station, which is a room that's just four plain

white walls where we can project images onto the walls; we can have audio with it; we can put text with it and make it like a film. We have that set up with all sorts of things on, but one of the most popular is just very gentle music and images of fish swimming in a pond. One of the men who attends the dementia café, when it gets too much for him, takes himself off and sits in there on his own and just watches it. When he's calm, he comes out again. So we have that breakout space which I think is really good.

(K. Morris, conversation with author, 22 November 2021)

Whilst few libraries may have the space or resources to install a separate sensory room, more may be able to draw on ideas from other sectors to create calm rooms (or calm corners) within the library that people with dementia – as well as people with other conditions – may find helpful to relax. For example, Crewe railway station in the UK has adapted a waiting room to provide a safe and calm environment. 'The Calm Corner' is a room that is specifically designed to offer customers, especially those with hidden disabilities, a safe and calm environment whilst waiting for their train. In contrast to the bright furnishing and lighting in the station's main waiting room, the calm corner features grey and green colours to give a calming effect; a 'living wall' of artificial greenery and plants; and specially designed comfortable furniture. There is LED rope lighting that changes brightness to suit those sitting in the space, as well as screens displaying historic images of Crewe (Granada, 2019).

Conclusion: maintaining dementia-friendly library design

I visited several dementia-friendly libraries whilst researching this book. Spending time in these libraries, it was clear that designers and architects had taken considerable care in the choices they made to try to ensure the buildings were accessible for people with dementia. However, it was also evident that the task of making sure a library is dementia friendly does not end once the designers leave. Whilst library staff cannot, of course, be expected to be experts in dementia-friendly design, it is important that all staff have a basic understanding of what makes a space dementia friendly and why certain features can be important to a person with dementia. Problems I observed in one or more libraries that are advertised as being dementia friendly included:

- cluttered, messy entrance areas
- dark-coloured mats on the floor (which may look like holes to some people with dementia)
- trip hazards (for example, bean bags in the middle of the room a similar colour to the floor)

- fold up chairs (rather than chairs with arms to make it easier to stand up) in areas where dementia-related resources are kept and likely to be used
- signage in shiny plastic holders, which can be difficult to read (rather than anti-glare alternatives)
- laminated signs in a glossy finish (rather than using matt laminator pouches, which are less likely to reflect light)
- potentially confusing noticeboards with *lots* of information flyers, but nothing to direct customers to the information they might be looking for (for example, sections for library information, local organisations, local events, etc.).

These observations – and the contrast in practices in libraries I visited – indicate the importance of staff understanding the reasoning behind design choices. There is little point in spending large sums of money on an impressive refurbishment if the good work is undermined by basic misunderstandings or oversights in the day-to-day operation of a library. On the other hand, knowledgeable staff can do a great deal to overcome any shortcomings in design and to capitalise on those features of the library building or layout that have the potential to make it more dementia friendly. The types of problems listed above also indicate areas that all libraries need to pay attention to, whether or not they have undergone a dementia-friendly refurbishment. All the examples listed could be improved at little or no cost. Not all libraries can afford new furnishings and décor, but all can make sure they remove clutter around entrances and have clearly labelled and well-organised noticeboards for example.

It is important that libraries involve people with dementia and their carers in decisions about changes to the library environment. For anyone interested in making improvements to the design of their library – even on a very informal basis – Chapter 9 offers suggestions on ways to involve people with dementia and carers in researching and evaluating library services, including buildings and environments. However, consultation should not simply be a one-off activity; there is undoubtedly value in asking for feedback on the library environment on a regular basis, especially to address the types of problems listed above that might creep into library practice but are relatively easy to fix.

Having discussed library design in detail, the following chapters move the focus onto resources and activities that take place within the library. Chapter 4 looks specifically at reading materials and reading-related activities.

4
Reading and Dementia

> If you're having a difficult day, if the person you care for is having a difficult day, if you feel you're not coping terribly well, sit down and read something together. It will take you right away from the here and now and into some other world that you can share and talk about.
>
> (Reading is Caring project evaluation interviewee)

There can sometimes be a perception that people with dementia are no longer able to take part in reading activities, but this is far from the case. In the early stages of dementia, many people continue to read by themselves and, even in the later stages, there are ways of making reading more accessible to people who no longer find it easy to read alone. Crucially, dementia can be an opportunity to expand what we mean when we talk about 'reading materials' or 'texts'. The basic definition of reading is the decoding of symbols to derive meaning. This means that reading materials can include not simply word-based materials, but also resources that we can 'read' in other ways and with other senses. This might include images and objects, movements and gestures or sounds and music that people with dementia may be able to make connections with.

This chapter starts with a caveat: reading is often suggested as a potentially beneficial activity for people with dementia and there are claims that it may lead to positive changes such as decreased agitation, reduced anxiety and depression and improved cognitive skills. However, robust research into literature interventions for people with dementia is currently limited, especially when compared to other arts and cultural interventions, such as music therapy. The research that does exist is often conflicting and indicates that any links between reading and possible 'improvements' in, or prevention of, dementia are complex and uncertain. To give just one example that illustrates some of these complexities, a study carried out in Japan found evidence that reading newspapers played a significant role in the decline of dementia symptoms, but oddly there was no similar change observed for reading books (Kim et al., 2016).

Research into the impacts of reading activities for people with dementia is at present limited and often contradictory. However, more convincing research is available into bibliotherapy more generally, that is, the use of books to help people to improve mental health and wellbeing. Research has established that reading has the potential to be relaxing, transportive and escapist (Brewster, 2017). It can also facilitate an emotional connection between a reader and a text (Cohen, 1992). In a group setting, the relationship between reading group members has a role to play, alongside the text itself, in establishing therapeutic outcomes such as increased confidence and social inclusion (Brewster, 2011; Dowrick et al., 2012; Longden et al., 2015). There is no reason to suppose that some, or all, of these potential benefits from reading might not equally apply to people with dementia. So, while more research is needed to determine whether, and how, reading has a role to play in helping to prevent or ameliorate the symptoms of dementia, we do know that, for many people, it can play an important role in supporting them to live well. This is illustrated through the case study examples in the latter sections of this chapter.

This chapter explores some of the ways in which libraries can offer reading activities for people with dementia and their carers. It starts by considering the importance of imagination and how this can be a powerful way to make connections with someone with dementia, potentially overriding memory problems they may be experiencing. It then highlights some examples of reading materials about dementia for a variety of audiences, as well as resources created specifically for people with dementia. The final section of the chapter presents case studies of activities intended to engage people with dementia, and in some cases their carers too, in reading. These include both group-based activities and one-to-one initiatives.

Dementia and imagination

As the writer Leslie Marmon Silko said, 'sometimes, what we call "memory" and what we call "imagination" are not so easily distinguished' (Silko, 2012, 227). That can be true for any of us, but it is particularly relevant for people with dementia. While dementia often results in problems with memory, this does not mean that a person's imagination is negatively impacted. In fact, people with dementia may draw on their imagination to fill gaps in their memory – just as most of us do from time to time. Memories and imagination become entangled and inseparable.

When my dad had dementia, the lines between what was real and what was a story often became blurred and, at times, the magical or imaginary were just as likely to be 'true' as real life. He would create stories to explain what was happening to him or how he was feeling. If I asked what he had been doing, for instance, he would be more likely to have 'been to Forge Lane' (the steelworks where he used to work) or 'been talking to Pop' (his father who died over 40 years before) than sitting in his room. Sometimes words or objects would get mixed up – so a bed would become a boat and a plastic bag would become a cat. But rather than being a problem, that opened up the possibility to tell stories and imagine what would happen if his bed really were a boat. Stories offer new ways of seeing things, and new ways of talking about things, which do not rely on memory. Dementia is often described as a 'shutting off' or 'closing down', but another way to think about it is as providing a way of playing with language and opening up the world of shared stories. Stories are, above all, a means of communicating – and to communicate, you need to accept certain conventions and shared meanings. It is easy to break the magic and expose a story as untrue, but instead we can choose to build a story together that lets us share experiences and feelings once more.

Internal and external texts

The notion of 'internal' and 'external' texts, as described by the Argentinian writer Laura Devetach (2010), can be helpful when developing reading interventions for people with dementia. According to Devetach, internal texts belong to our personal world; they are texts that have impacted on us in some way and continue to intercede in our lives. These might be complete texts, such as a novel; but alternatively, they may be fragments of poems, stories or songs (or simply words or phrases that we do not remember clearly) that in one way or another continue to intervene in our lives. External texts, on the other hand, belong to the collective world and give us a sense of belonging to a group.

Often, people with dementia retain a rich library of internal texts: songs they remember; poems they learnt at school; idioms or dialect expressions; or familiar stories and rhymes. However, these are often not exploited as effectively as they could be as a way of making connections with people with dementia. I witnessed an example of how drawing on internal texts can work successfully in one of the sessions I observed for the Words in Mind project (described below). In a reading group session in a care home, a discussion of texts about birds prompted one of the participants to start singing the nursery rhyme 'Sing a Song of Sixpence' (for lyrics see www.poetryfoundation.org/poems/42900/sing-a-song-of-sixpence), an internal text that he could clearly remember from an earlier stage of his life. The facilitator immediately responded by encouraging the whole group to join in singing the nursery rhyme, transforming the participant's internal text into an external one that could be enjoyed by the whole group.

Dementia-friendly reading materials

Having outlined some ideas that can help to inform the provision of reading experiences for, and with, people with dementia, the next section explores the types of reading materials that can be effective. This discussion is split into two sections: the first looks explicitly at resources *about* dementia itself, which can be targeted at a variety of audiences, whilst the second section discusses reading materials, of varied formats and on a range of topics, that may be particularly suitable *for* people with dementia.

Resources about dementia

Resources about dementia can include materials for a range of audiences depending on the customer base of a library: people with dementia themselves; their carers, family and friends; health and social care practitioners or students and others with a professional interest in the topic; children and young people, especially those who may have a parent or grandparent with dementia; and members of the general public who may simply want to know more about dementia or perhaps are concerned about someone they know. The following are examples of some of the schemes and initiatives that help to identify resources about dementia and make them more easily accessible to library customers.

It is worth mentioning that reviewing dementia resource identification and recognition schemes, such as those described below, highlighted the dearth of materials about the condition written specifically for people with dementia themselves. In contrast to most other health conditions, relatively few resources about dementia are written with people living with the condition in mind. This can obviously present challenges for library staff if they are asked for resources to help people who have dementia to better understand their condition.

Reading Well Books on Prescription for Dementia

Many libraries in the UK stock titles from The Reading Agency's 'Reading Well Books on Prescription for Dementia' scheme. The scheme is part of the wider national Reading Well Books on Prescription programme, which provides book-based support to people living with a range of conditions, including adults with common mental health conditions; children and young people experiencing difficulties with mental health and wellbeing; and people with long-term health conditions and their carers (The Reading Agency, 2022). The Books on Prescription model was first developed in Wales in 2005 by Professor Neil Frude and was adopted across England in 2013. Under this scheme, users either receive a recommendation of a title from a health or social care professional or can self-refer to the scheme by simply visiting a library.

The Reading Agency and the Society of Chief Librarians (now Libraries Connected) developed the first Books on Prescription list for people with dementia and their carers in 2015 with the support of a wide range of partners from health and social care sectors. At the initial stage of development, an external consultant wrote a consultation paper that considered the key areas of need and the policy and evidence base underpinning the scheme (The Reading Agency and Society of Chief Librarians, 2013). To gain consensus on the priorities for the scheme, the consultation paper was circulated to relevant professional health bodies and experts including the Alzheimer's Society, the British Psychological Society, Innovations in Dementia CIC and the Royal College of Psychiatrists. Representatives from these organisations then helped to develop the book list, drawing on their breadth and depth of knowledge and understanding of dementia and dementia care.

Books on the list are divided into the following categories: information and advice; support for living well; advice for relatives and carers; and personal stories. The book selection process aimed to provide a balance of non-fiction, fiction and memoir titles. The list includes items specially designed to support people with lower reading levels and learning disabilities, and carers for whom English is an additional language. The information and advice section of the list includes information on normal ageing and memory problems; general information about dementia; and a title suitable for children. The texts range from academic works to more accessible books. There are resources aimed at health and social care professionals, as well as at families, carers and the general public. The advice for relatives and carers section covers both practical and emotional support for carers and families of people with dementia, for example with practicalities and relationships; information on medications and types of therapy; how to access additional help and services; and the financial and legal aspects of caring for someone with dementia. The living well with dementia section includes activities and books to share between people with dementia and their families and carers, as well as advice on issues such as finance and communication. The inclusion of fiction and personal stories about dementia was a new development for this list that has since been replicated in other aspects of the Reading Well Books on Prescription programme. For a more detailed description of the development of Reading Well Books on Prescription for Dementia, see Walworth (2018).

The Reading Well Books on Prescription collection is a useful starting point for libraries wanting to offer books about dementia within their collection. However, it is important to be aware that the books included vary considerably in terms of accessibility and target audience. Importantly, in contrast to other Reading Well Books on Prescription lists that focus on self-help titles, many of the books on the dementia list are likely to be inaccessible to many people with dementia themselves. More explicit information about who a book is aimed at, who it is written by (for example, healthcare professional, academic, carer, person with dementia, journalist) and level of existing knowledge or general reading level required could help not only members of the public, but also library staff who may want to recommend books to customers.

This emphasises the point that libraries need to offer guidance to customers, as well as making books and other resources about dementia available. Whilst this can happen on an informal basis, the 'Dementia Australia staff recommend sticker' demonstrates one way of formalising this process.

Dementia Australia staff recommend sticker

To assist users in navigating their library collection, Dementia Australia has developed a 'Dementia Australia staff recommend sticker'. The organisation has a collection of over 14,000 items, so they recognise the importance of assisting users in finding resources. The recommended sticker strategy is based on the 'staff picks' approach many people are familiar with seeing in their local bookshop.

Resources meeting the criteria for the sticker need to:

- be well-written or well-produced
- use positive language
- consistently receive good feedback from borrowers
- have positive reviews from specialist clinicians
- have broad appeal according to library staff.

This simple strategy has been helpful for volunteer staff, as well as for library users, particularly at times when library staff are not available. The library service sends out pop-up libraries to social events such as memory cafés. The pop-up is staffed by volunteers who use the stickers to assist selections for new users.

The sticker currently only applies to the library's physical collection, but more recently Dementia Australia has started developing online library guides to assist users in navigating a range of curated digital resources by subject. These guides include e-books, journal articles, video content, websites and apps. In the future, the organisation is planning to use QR codes on book covers to link users to relevant online guides for related resources (S. Mauritzen, e-mail to author, 8 November 2021).

Knowledge hubs for health and social care professionals
Whilst public libraries are most likely to focus on resources for people with dementia and their carers, health and academic libraries naturally need to provide resources for those working, or studying to work, in health or social care. As the majority of resources for this audience are usually in a digital format rather than print, this often involves curating a set of resources in a variety of media and from different sources and making them available to library users from a single portal page. An example is East Cheshire NHS Trust Library and Knowledge Service (2021), which provides a number of online Condition Knowledge Hubs with links to information on specific topics, including dementia. This hub includes books on dementia in the library catalogue; evidence resources such as the Cochrane Library of systematic reviews; links to relevant organisations, websites and training resources; current awareness services; social media; apps; and the library's 'health stories' collection of personal stories about living with health conditions.

Resources for children and young people
Another audience that is worth briefly highlighting is children and young people. A number of organisations provide lists of books about dementia for young people, especially those who may have a grandparent or other relative diagnosed with dementia. In the UK, BookTrust (2019) has a list of resources that may be helpful for children and young people. As well as a short synopsis of each title, there is information about the appropriate reading age and interest age for each book to guide library staff, or other adults, wishing to recommend a book to a young person. There are also reader reviews of the

books listed. Similarly, the HealthyBooks (2022) website has a section on books to support children and young people affected by dementia. For each title, there is a short review and an indication of the age group it is likely to be appropriate for.

Reactions to resources about dementia

This section has highlighted some of the resources available that may be useful for libraries wishing to add materials about dementia to their collection. However, staff working with customers should be mindful that certain narratives or ideas about dementia can produce strong reactions – and often not in ways that might be anticipated. Of course, libraries should not censor materials or stop people from borrowing potentially challenging titles, but staff need to be aware that people with dementia – and possibly other customers too – may sometimes find resources about dementia challenging to read.

An example that illustrates the need to consider how people may react to certain texts occurred when I shared a selection of comics and graphic narratives about experiences of dementia (many of them highly regarded and award nominees/winners) with a peer support group for people living with dementia. Group members criticised the overly negative themes and content of many of the examples shared, which they felt did not correspond to their own experiences of living with dementia. An example was *Tangles*, an award-winning graphic novel written by Sarah Leavitt that tells the story of her mother's experience of Alzheimer's disease and the resulting impact on her family. Leavitt writes, 'It gets hard to see someone as a person when they've become a list of needs' (Leavitt, 2012, 85). She also shows this as being her mother's view of herself on occasions: for example, when her mother says '"I'm a nobody! I'm not a real person anymore!"' (Leavitt, 2012, 67), and, later in the story, '"I'm not really much of a person right now"' (Leavitt, 2012, 98) alongside a blank silhouette of her image. In contrast, members of the peer support group commented on ways in which their lives had many positive elements – a message they felt was missing from this story and from many of the other graphic narratives I shared with them. They felt that the ways in which people with dementia were portrayed encouraged readers to view them differently, as abnormal or perhaps even less than human. For a fuller description of the peer support group's reactions to a range of titles, see McNicol and Leamy (2020).

Of course, this sort of reaction does not mean that *Tangles* should not be stocked in libraries. Indeed, other people with dementia, as well as carers, will likely be able to empathise with Leavitt's story and feel it reflects their own situation and feelings. However, it does highlight the importance of having opportunities to discuss reactions to books about, and portrayals of, dementia. In the situation described above, there were dementia advocates supporting the session and we decided on a positive outcome – to create a comic that the group felt more accurately reflected their experiences (see Chapter 5). However, this experience illustrates the need to be aware that resources about dementia can produce strong reactions and to be prepared for these.

General reading materials for people with dementia

As mentioned above, there are, unfortunately, relatively few resources about dementia written explicitly for people with dementia themselves. However, there are many examples of reading materials on more general topics that can be used by, and with, people with dementia.

The types of texts that are appropriate for individuals will, naturally, differ depending on many factors, including their interests, previous reading experiences and the ways in which they are affected by dementia. In general, however, shorter texts with relatively simple sentences are often helpful. However, this suggestion is not as straightforward as it might at first sound. For example, 'easy readers' – simplified stories for people learning a language or with special educational needs – are usually not shortened in a way that is most helpful for people with dementia. In contrast to the majority of target audiences for easy reader titles, it is often the complexity of the story, rather than the language itself, that proves most problematic for people with dementia. Children's books are an option that can work well for some people, especially if they have a particular significance – perhaps titles people remember from their childhood or stories they shared with their own children or grandchildren. However, children's books more generally can often feel patronising if they are presented to an adult reader with dementia.

The examples below illustrate some of the types of reading resources available specifically for people with dementia. Whilst this section draws on particular examples to provide a detailed description of how this type of resource can be helpful for someone with dementia, in all cases there are other organisations that produce similar resources.

Picture books

Pictures to Share books are found in many libraries in the UK and more widely. These are large, glossy picture books designed to engage and entertain people with mid- to late-stage dementia and to promote meaningful and enjoyable communication with friends, family and carers. Importantly, Pictures to Share books do not look like children's picture books; they are more like adult coffee table books. The books include images, song lyrics and well-known poems in large print on a particular theme, such as family life, gardens or pets. A person with dementia can interpret what they see in the books in a variety of ways; they may respond with words, facial expressions or by touching the page, for example. The publisher has produced a guide to help carers use the books effectively (Pictures to Share, n.d.).

Heather Rodenhurst, Team Librarian from Shropshire Libraries in the UK, describes how she has witnessed readers responding to Pictures to Share books:

> The books were immediately really popular because they are so visual and interactive. You could literally take any page and most people would see something in the picture, or something in the quote or some lyric that would immediately prompt a memory or prompt them to say something or perhaps remember the poem that it came from.
>
> (H. Rodenhurst, conversation with author, 9 November 2021)

Simplified texts

Dovetale Press (2016), based in New Zealand, has created versions of 'classic' stories, such as *Little Women* and *A Christmas Carol*, in which text that is not essential to the stories has been removed, shortening the novels considerably and simplifying the plot. However, in contrast to most 'easy reader' versions of these types of texts, the Dovetale Press versions retain the authors' original language as far as possible. This is something that may be particularly appealing to someone who has read the novel previously, so might find the language familiar. All the books include illustrations, some of which were included in the original publications. The pages are designed so that each double page can be read as a single entity, which means that even if a person cannot remember what happened on the previous pages, reading can still be a pleasurable experience. There are 'cast lists' for each novel and, where appropriate, a summary is provided after every chapter as a reminder of the storyline.

Step-by-step books

Many resources for people with dementia focus on compensating for memory problems, but it is also important to consider resources for people affected by dementia in other ways. For example, people with dementia can often find it difficult to carry out a sequence of activities, so following a recipe, for instance, can become challenging. There are relatively few examples of step-by-step resources specifically for people with dementia, but books designed for people with learning disabilities may be useful. An example is a series of *Cook and Eat* cookbooks – step-by-step guides to preparing basic dishes, with pictures of ingredients, cutlery and utensils needed for cooking, with timings included, so that people can focus on doing the instructions one at a time (South West Yorkshire Partnership NHS Foundation Trust, 2022).

Shared memory bags, Shropshire Libraries, UK

As emphasised above, books or written resources are not the only type of texts or reading materials available for people with dementia. 'Texts' can also include objects, images, sounds and so forth. Many public library services offer reminiscence kits suitable for people with dementia. However, the shared memory bags created by Shropshire Libraries (n.d.) in the UK take a slightly different approach. These are based around the Pictures to Share books (described above), offering a set of reading-related resources that might stimulate memories, but equally can prompt imaginative responses.

Each shared memory bag is a portable collection of objects, books and activities to share either one-to-one or in a group to prompt conversation. The memory bags can be borrowed from the public library free of charge. Themes available include school days, football, seaside, pets, shopping, childhood, travel and the countryside. The 'In the Garden' memory bag, for example, includes a wildflowers album, cloth daisy chain, tree card game, 'types of flower' poster, flower memory game, sweet pea candle, artificial flowers and a user guide with conversation starters.

Heather Rodenhurst, Team Librarian from Shropshire Libraries, describes how the shared memory bag scheme was developed, building on a more reminiscence-focused project:

> The beginning of the project came about in 2013 when our Health and Wellbeing Librarian began a project with Shropshire Museums. They created five memory bags. Each was in a laptop bag and had a theme, like school days, football and time for tea. Working together, the library and museum staff sourced objects that fitted those themes, were tactile and would appeal to all the senses. They created a booklet with laminated sheets that would give a bit of information about each artefact and also some memory prompts. Because the museum service was involved, there was an emphasis on the history of the object and how it had developed. People were able to borrow a bag using their library card and it proved really popular.

Building on this, we decided that we would like to extend our memory bag collection, but we would base the bags around a book – because we're libraries, so that makes sense! We realised that care settings would likely want to borrow these, but I was also thinking about the huge number of carers who are at home day after day having to fill those long hours, not just with practical care, but with therapeutic or distracting activities, and who might not know where to start. So, we went through a Pictures to Share book and for every page in the book, we came up with some conversation prompts. We included objects on the theme in each bag as well. We bear in mind that the objects that go into the memory bags must be as durable as possible because they're going to be handled multiple times. Plus, we don't want the overall weight of the bag to be more than your average carer could pick up and carry.

We find that the childhood days bag is very popular. We've got a couple of sporting life bags and they can be very appealing to men in particular. We created a bilingual Welsh-English pack based around the bilingual Pictures to Share book. That was funded by Welsh language groups here in Oswestry, which is on the border so has a Welsh-speaking community. That bag is popular because I don't think there's anything else that replicates that kind of activity. We also had some funding from the Diocese of Lichfield to create a couple of bags for 'Strength for the Journey', a faith-based Pictures to Share book. We have one in the library and we created a duplicate for one of the local churches to use with members of their congregation. Those have been well used.

We've used volunteer help to create the packs. My branch library has a history of using student help and having placements for young people who are struggling to get into work. So, we've used that help to create the guides for the shared memory bags. Usually, myself or another member of staff will go through the book first and make a note of what we think the prompts should be. Then a volunteer will put it together in the standard format. We wanted a standardised look so that people would know what they were getting each time. We've done tranches of five or six bags at a time as and when we could get a little bit of funding – a lot of it has been produced on very small amounts of funding.

We bought packaging materials as well because we have to try and make sure that the objects we've invested this public money in remain in as good a condition as possible and that they withstand multiple trips around the county. So, they all have safe packaging and that helps us to manage hygiene issues as well.

We have a system of staff guidelines so that when bags come back, staff can check them through. Every user guide has a contents page on the front so staff have a checklist of what should be in the pack. It also means people using them at home have a checklist to make sure they put all the contents back in the bag before they return it.

(H. Rodenhurst, conversation with author, 9 November 2021)

In addition to the shared memory bags, Shropshire Libraries has developed the Oswestry Memory Loss Collection, an expanded range of resources to support those living with memory loss at home, including jigsaw puzzles, games, fidget widgets, sensory sound CDs and reminiscence picture cards. Having items such as these available to loan gives carers (or people with dementia themselves) an opportunity to try out different resources, perhaps before buying items that they find work particularly well. The collection also includes specialist books about dementia that may not be found in the general collection, for example, titles about sex and wellbeing, yoga and nutrition and hydration (Shropshire Libraries, n.d.). Items for this collection were selected in consultation with local dementia day groups and a member of the Local Dementia Action Alliance (see Chapter 7).

Reading activities for people with dementia and carers

Of course, making reading materials available for people to borrow and read at home is only part of a library's role; many libraries also offer reading activities for customers. Carers often take part in library reading groups to give themselves a respite from caring responsibilities and some libraries run dedicated carers' reading groups. These are often supported by local carer support organisations and have a focus on sharing experiences with people in a similar situation, as well as enjoying literature. For example, as part of the Artful Age programme, managed by Durham County Council Community Arts Team in the UK, a Reading Together group was set up in October 2020, at a time when many COVID-19 restrictions remained in place in the UK. This online group ran until April 2022 when restrictions on face-to-face meetings had been lifted. Selected reading material was posted out to participants from across East Durham a week in advance under instructions not to open the envelope until the start of the online session. Whilst not all participants were carers, feedback from someone who was caring for her mother (who has dementia) described how attending the sessions allowed her to have some 'me time' (C. Robson, e-mail to author, 22 April 2022). (Online activities for carers, as well as people with dementia, are discussed in greater detail in Chapter 6.)

In recent years there has been an increasing awareness of the value of creative arts practice in dementia care and, as a result, growing interest in expanding bibliotherapy services to engage with people living with dementia. Sometimes a person with dementia, especially if they are in the early stages of the condition, will take part in a general reading group within the library. In these instances, the advice on communication strategies in Chapter 2 may be helpful to ensure that everyone is able to participate in the group effectively. However, as their condition progresses, or perhaps if they feel less confident, specific reading initiatives designed for people with dementia can often be helpful. Carers may also attend these groups to support the person they are caring for. In most cases these initiatives do not require people to read themselves – although they may do so if they so wish. The types of reading activities for people with dementia described below can help people to continue to read even if they struggle to follow a printed text on their own, by, for example, someone reading to them or through reading together.

Group reading activities

Group reading activities are probably the most common form of reading initiative for people with dementia offered in libraries, although some schemes include both group and one-to-one options. The following section outlines a number of group reading activities used in libraries, or in similar community settings. These examples demonstrate a variety of approaches that can be taken.

Shared Reading

Probably the most well-known approach to group bibliotherapy activities is that led by The Reader organisation in Liverpool in the UK, which has created a 'Shared Reading' model that works with people to increase their appreciation of classic fiction and poetry. This model has spread throughout the world, including Australasia, Scandinavia and North America. Originally working with people with mental health problems, The Reader also works with people with dementia. Their model predominantly uses literary works that they describe as 'great literature'. Shared Reading groups for people with dementia are typically shorter than standard sessions, running for a maximum of one hour and using shorter materials such as short stories and poems rather than entire novels. Varied facilitation techniques are used, based on the needs and abilities of participants. With individuals who have dementia, the facilitator might spend more time describing a poem or talk in a louder voice, for instance, depending on the specific needs of the group. Participants are welcome to share their experiences and reminisce, but the focus is on enjoying the literature itself (Longden et al., 2016).

Dawn DeVries and colleagues conducted a systematic review of research into Shared Reading groups for older adults with dementia. The five research studies they reviewed describe a variety of benefits and outcomes to individuals who participated in the sessions. Identified benefits included improved social engagement and interaction; enhanced quality of life;

improved relationships with other group members, staff, family members and other residents of their care home; improved mood and behaviour; a sense of enjoyment expressed by participants and observed by staff and family; improved communication; creating a sense of identify; opportunities for self-expression; and increased appropriateness of comments and conversation. However, the reviewers noted that an adaptation that appeared to be missing from the research on Shared Reading was the use of props and visual stimuli to assist in setting the stage and to create a sensorimotor experience; in this model, the focus is very much on what we would traditionally think of as a 'text' (DeVries et al., 2019).

Tales and Travel Memories

Tales and Travel Memories is a book and reading programme for people with Alzheimer's disease and related dementias. It was designed by retired academic librarian Mary Beth Riedner and Gail Borden Public Library District staff and volunteers in Illinois in the US. The programme is delivered at assisted living facilities in Elgin, Illinois, by volunteers and library staff. Each one-hour session takes participants on an imaginary trip to another country or another region of the US and includes books, music, objects, folktales and interesting facts about each destination country or region. In contrast to the Shared Reading technique described above, Tales and Travel Memories has a multi-sensory approach, making use of supplementary materials, including music, artefacts from the destination, colouring pages and even food. A typical session involves participants taking turns reading aloud from a folktale or story representative of the area; reading aloud interesting facts about the region (typed in a large, clear font); browsing illustrated books about the destination from the library's adult and children's collections; and taking part in informal conversations.

Travelling kits in suitcases are also available to borrow from the public library. Kits include several non-fiction books about a destination, examples of music, a DVD and other items. The check-out kits are designed to provide a similar experience to group sessions, but in a one-on-one setting. This enables carers to engage with the people with dementia they care for in new ways, to stimulate conversation and reminisce. The Tales and Travel Memories website also contains a free toolbox with a selection of 'excursion guides' and adapted versions of traditional folktales (Tales and Travel, n.d.).

Words in Mind

Third Sector Leaders Kirklees, an organisation that manages a number of volunteer schemes, ran a bibliotherapy scheme called Words in Mind between 2018 and 2021. Words in Mind built on a longer history of bibliotherapy in Kirklees. Kirklees public library service was innovative in being the only public library service in the UK to employ bibliotherapists with a specific remit to deliver group sessions. This role was dissolved in 2016 and it became part of the librarians' outreach work. Words in Mind evolved from this history of bibliotherapy and worked alongside the public library service to deliver bibliotherapy across the district. Words in Mind was delivered by volunteers and sessional workers trained to run reading groups for people with dementia and/or people experiencing mental health problems. Groups ran in various locations, including residential care homes, hospital wards, public libraries and as part of established community groups, such as a social group for people with young-onset dementia. I was involved in research into this initiative, together with a colleague (Brewster and McNicol, 2019).

The direction of a Words in Mind group was shaped by the group members and tailored to their needs and interests, under the guidance of a group facilitator. The project adopted a person-centred approach and the starting point in planning a session was the needs of participants rather than the literature or other texts used. Responding to participants' interests and requirements meant that some groups shared the task of reading aloud, while others relied on the facilitator to read poems and prose to the group. In some groups substantial time was given over to sharing personal experiences in relation to the texts, while others focused more on the content of the resources shared and left less time for reflection. This led to a clear sense of 'ownership' for participants; the group belonged to them and could be shaped by their needs.

Most Words in Mind sessions made use of a wide variety of texts and resources. These varied from session to session, but commonly included 'classic' or well-known books and poems; lesser-known texts; 'popular' texts (for example, funny poems); lyrics; quotes; images; sensory resources (things to smell or touch); newspaper and magazine articles; local history resources; short stories or quick reads; and (auto)biographies. Facilitators did not place literary value judgements on the resources selected; their value was solely determined by the extent to which they encouraged engagement within the group. Sessions in care homes typically included a range of media, such as images, objects/props, large print books, picture books and reminiscence resources – being mindful to balance the need to provide stimulus without being overwhelming and ensuring objects were suitable for the group.

Words in Mind therefore focused on the use of different media and types of resource within sessions for people with dementia. This makes its approach markedly different from models such as Shared Reading, which places strong emphasis on the importance of written texts, only recommending visual imagery and song to 'help those who cannot follow the reading material' (Billington et al., 2013, 21). This might mean that a Words in Mind session included games and singing for instance, or simple activities like the creation of a 'memory jar'. Facilitators also made use of objects, particularly those that might stimulate a range of senses, for example flowers to smell, pebbles to touch or fruit to taste.

Participants in Words in Mind sessions could decide how they wished to contribute to a session and all contributions were valued. For participants with dementia, simply being aware and making eye contact during the session could be an important outcome of taking part. Amongst people living with dementia, some of the texts might bring a sense of recognition and stimulate memories, for example about poems they had learnt at school.

It was not simply about making connections with the past, however; the main outcomes for participants with dementia were seen in terms of conversation and promoting social interaction through connections made with the various texts. A sense of calm and relaxation was another important therapeutic benefit of Words in Mind groups for many participants. Relaxation was a key impact for those who participated in the groups, particularly in those care homes where few other relaxing activities took place. There was also evidence of longer-term impacts of Words in Mind. Some participants appeared to recall the emotion of a session, if not specific details, for example, by remaining less agitated afterwards or appearing pleased to see the facilitator again. In common with other arts-related activities, for some care home residents, participating in Words in Mind sessions highlighted individual talents, such as singing ability, which care home staff had not been aware of previously.

There was a feeling amongst some volunteers who facilitated Words in Mind groups in different locations that participants in the community mental health groups 'seem to bring more to the session', for example by bringing along their own writing or taking turns to read, whereas in care homes, 'they're very happy to listen'. As another facilitator described, in a care home, 'it's almost like you're performing'. This highlights an important point: facilitating a reading group for people with dementia is likely to differ in certain ways from facilitating similar activities for other groups of participants. Volunteers or staff are likely to need additional support and training to help them to support participants, including being aware that participants may be actively involved in alternative ways. Participants in care home groups did, in fact, bring their own contributions to the sessions, but they did so a little differently than might be the case in other groups; for example, by spontaneously singing or reciting rather than preparing something to bring along in advance.

Table 4.1 shows how the outcomes of Words in Mind for people with dementia can be mapped onto Tom Kitwood's model, which was described in Chapter 1. This demonstrates how the sessions were underpinned by a person-centred approach. Thinking about the outcomes of reading- or library-based activities in this way can be helpful when working in partnership with professionals from health and social care sectors as it presents the activities in terms that they are likely to be familiar with (See Chapter 7).

Table 4.1 *Outcomes of Words in Mind mapped onto Kitwood's model*

Attachment	People make connections to each other and to shared texts (which in turn may connect them to memories or people from earlier in their lives).
Comfort	The sessions offer an opportunity for relaxation. Some people appeared less agitated after a session and were pleased to see the facilitator again.
Inclusion	People living with dementia feel more included and able to play a valued part in activities and relationships, through members of the group reading together, for example, and all contributions being valued and, as far as possible, incorporated into the session.
Identity	Reading materials and approaches are tailored around the identities and interests of the group. Individual group members are encouraged to input with their own memories and reactions.
Occupation	Words in Mind offers people an enjoyable, stimulating and accessible activity with various ways for people to become involved (for example, listening, reading, singing, touching/smelling/tasting objects, talking).

For a more detailed description of the research into Words in Mind, see Brewster and McNicol (2021).

Montessori book clubs

Yet another approach to reading groups – and one that offers a contrast to Words in Mind – is dementia book clubs based on Montessori principles. Dementia the Montessori Way run book clubs based on approaches devised by Maria Montessori. Although these techniques are most commonly used in early years settings, this organisation has adapted and adjusted these principles to support people with dementia. The clubs, predominantly in care settings rather than the community, are facilitated by staff or family members and are a place for people with dementia to enjoy conversation and company. Some of the clubs achieve specific goals, such as reading a certain amount, while others simply offer stimulation. The approach is based on principles of invitation, courtesy and grace (Bracken, 2020).

As with Shared Reading, there is a strong focus on written text, but rather than stressing the value of 'classic' literature, this approach uses books written especially for people with dementia. The style, content and layout of the set of UK-targeted books has been inspired by the books written in the series *Carry on Reading in Dementia* by Gail Elliot for DementiaAbility, Canada (https://dementiability.com). The books are intended to be 'straightforward but not patronising' (Bracken, 2020). The appearance of the writing, its size and how it is laid out on the page have been tested with groups and individuals. Assessing a person's ability to read before they join a group is important in this approach, along with inviting people to come to the club. Typically, each group member reads a page (the words 'next reader please' appear at the bottom of each page). Each page contains two or three simple, factual sentences on a discrete topic. Many pages also include a question to prompt conversation – these are usually closed questions (requiring yes/no answers). The books do not contain what proponents of this approach describe as 'distracting' pictures. This means that, for instance, a page from *1970s – The Pivot of Change* (Elliot, 2020) discussing Michael Jackson's *Off the Wall* album has three short sentences and a question, but does not include any images of either the singer or album cover. This approach therefore relies on readers with dementia being able to remember, or relate to, the words rather than being prompted to make comments or recollections in response to supporting images.

One-to-one reading

Whilst a number of libraries run reading groups for people with dementia, there is also a need for one-to-one activities, in particular for people who are housebound or live in more isolated areas without easy access to a library or other community venue, or who simply prefer a one-to-one setting.

Reading is Caring

Reading is Caring, run by the national charity Scottish Book Trust, is based on the notion that shared reading can help a person with dementia and their carer (which could be a family member, friend or paid carer) to maintain their relationship, as well as helping the carer to find ways to join their loved one on their unique dementia journey and, through personal reading, find some respite from stress that may be caused by their caring responsibilities (Scottish Book Trust, 2022). This approach is particularly interesting in that it aims to provide direct benefits for carers, as well as for people with dementia.

The aim of the Reading is Caring pilot project (2020–21) was to test a range of ways in which shared reading may be useful to people living with dementia and their carers. The programme offers training to carers on how to bring a shared reading approach into their relationship with the person they care for. The training covers practical techniques and person-centred approaches around components such as text selection; reading voice and pace; using illustration and sensory objects in parallel with reading; and asking questions. During the training sessions, carers have an opportunity to practise using a variety of shared reading materials, including short stories, poems, scripts, cartoons and non-fiction materials. They are also prompted to consider the variety of ways that these can be read, including: the carer reading aloud; the person with dementia reading aloud; reading together; taking turns to read; and choosing texts that encourage repetition or call and response. The training also covers making life story book boxes. These are similar to memory boxes but include reading materials that are likely to be meaningful to the person with dementia, in addition to objects, images and so forth usually found in a memory box. Carers are then encouraged and supported to build regular shared reading into their relationship with the person living with dementia. The training was originally intended to be delivered in face-to-face workshops, but due to the COVID-19 pandemic, sessions were moved to online delivery on either a one-to-one or small group basis (see Chapter 6). Alongside colleagues, I was involved in an evaluation of this pilot (McNicol and Dalton, 2021).

For people who are not used to reading aloud on a regular basis, and who may not have been asked to do so since they were at school, the act of reading out loud can feel intimidating at first. Several carers commented on how taking part in the Reading is Caring workshops had helped them to overcome their initial hesitancy and gain confidence through suggestions such as reading slowly, pre-reading material before they share it and making use of illustrations.

Carers who took part in workshops described how Reading is Caring has the potential to impact on caring relationships as members of the family came together to support the shared reading process. This might involve a person with dementia and their carer creating a life story book box together, for instance, or involving children or grandchildren in its creation. For care staff, the links between the Reading is Caring approach and life story work, especially the creation of life story book boxes, made it easier for them to think about ways of integrating shared reading with existing approaches they might adopt when working with someone with dementia. An individual's life story book box, or favourite books, could be shared with care staff to help them to better understand the life and interests of the person with dementia or to help other relatives to engage more effectively.

Carers described how they had witnessed the shared reading process appear to bring comfort to the person they were caring for, often in particularly distressing situations. As a carer said, reading together acted as 'a really good de-stressor' when both they and the person with dementia might be finding things difficult. Shared reading was also reported to bring comfort and aid relaxation in everyday situations and often this effect appeared to last long beyond the reading period itself.

There was also evidence from the pilot phase that Reading is Caring has positive benefits for carers' own mental health and wellbeing. Carers appreciated the suggestion of finding reading materials that were of interest, not only to the person with dementia, but for them too. They spoke about the shared reading experience being a relaxing one for both parties. It was not simply the act of reading itself that was relaxing, but also the knowledge that they were doing something positive that might be stimulating, or comforting, for the person they were caring for.

The pilot found that, through shared reading, some people may respond to things they were interested in in the past, but others might be more focused on things that are important to them in the present. Shared reading might also help a person with dementia to share aspects of their identity, such as activities they enjoy or places they had visited, with a carer. For carers who had not known the person earlier in their life, this could help them to get a richer picture of who they were (and are) as a person. Even amongst carers who knew a person with dementia well, shared reading, as well as being a stimulating activity in itself, could lead on to further discussions, reflections and other forms of stimulation.

Table 4.2 shows how the outcomes of Reading is Caring for people with dementia can be mapped onto Tom Kitwood's model, which was described in Chapter 1. This demonstrates how Reading is Caring is underpinned by a person-centred approach.

Table 4.2 *Outcomes of Reading is Caring for people with dementia mapped onto Kitwood's model*

Attachment	Reading is Caring has the potential to support people living with dementia to have relationships based on genuine partnership and to feel close to others.
Comfort	The process aids relaxation and helps to relieve stress in difficult situations.
Inclusion	People living with dementia feel more included and able to play a valued part in activities and relationships (for example, both reading together). It places relationships on a more equal footing (rather than being based on 'carer' and 'cared for').
Identity	Reading materials and approaches are tailored around the identity and interests of the person with dementia.
Occupation	It offers people an enjoyable, stimulating and accessible activity that can take place easily alongside other activities, such as cooking or eating.

Although Reading is Caring is not specifically a library-based activity, the evaluation of the pilot phase provides evidence for, and helps to demonstrate, some of the potential benefits of reading activities for people with dementia and for their carers too (McNicol and Dalton, 2021). The idea of supporting the creation of life story book boxes, for instance, could certainly be of relevance to library staff. The approach taken in Reading is Caring could be valuable for facilitators of reading groups, as well as for one-to-one activities, as it suggests alternative ways of reading with people with dementia that enables them to take a more equal role in the activity.

Conclusions

This chapter has highlighted a number of considerations in relation to reading resources and activities for people with dementia and their carers. Firstly, the fact that 'reading' can have a broader definition than we might normally consider (for example, include a wider range of resources, not just word-based materials) and can use a variety of approaches depending on the needs and interests of those involved. The use of sensory objects is becoming increasingly common, but these are still mainly used as a support or enhancement for a reading experience based around written texts. There is scope for greater awareness and use of non-word-based resources, including objects, images, sounds and movements, as 'texts' that can be read (or decoded) in their own right. Some of the arts-based activities described in Chapter 5 suggest ways in which this might start to take place, thus opening up reading experiences further. This illustrates the importance of library staff sharing knowledge, both within the sector and beyond, to help them to make decisions about approaches to engage customers with dementia in reading activities.

The possibilities for reading (in its broadest definition) is an area where libraries have an important role to play in developing our understanding of, and responses to, dementia. Whilst museum and archive services, for instance, draw on their inherent strengths to support reminiscence activities, libraries' most obvious strength relates the role of imagination – stimulated through all forms of 'reading'. This links back to the discussion at the start of this chapter about the connections between imagination and memory. Whilst reminiscence resources and activities are primarily intended to stimulate memories, many texts provided via library services are created to prompt imaginative responses. The value of imagination should not be under-estimated; asking for imaginative responses, rather than memories, can take pressure off those struggling to recall facts and can mean some with dementia are more willing to engage. By emphasising what remains as a strength for many people, even those with more advanced dementia, reading can be a crucial part of a dementia-positive approach in which libraries have a central role to play.

Whilst reading is likely to remain at the centre of most libraries' offer for people with dementia, Chapter 5 looks at other types of activities for people with dementia and their carers that libraries can also support. This includes therapeutic activities, events to encourage social interaction and arts-based activities.

5
Health, Social and Arts Activities

> Connection is the key and anything that facilitates that connection is prioritised.
> (Sara Griffiths, The National Archives, UK, in e-mail to author)

Chapter 4 focused on reading-related resources and activities that libraries might offer for people with dementia and their carers. This chapter considers a wider range of activities that libraries might also provide. Broadly speaking, these fit under three themes: health-related or therapeutic initiatives; activities emphasising the importance of social connections; and arts-related activities that encourage involvement in a variety of art and cultural activities. Each of these three areas is underpinned by a distinct set of research literature that explains how and why these activities might be helpful for someone with dementia. Some of this research is outlined briefly within each section and, for each of the three themes, there are a number of examples and case studies illustrating the types of practical activities that libraries can offer. Activities specifically for people with dementia are of course important, but libraries also need to consider adjustments that can be made to enable people with dementia to join in activities aimed at a broader population. As far as possible, both approaches are reflected in the case studies described.

Health and therapy-informed activities

The first theme covers activities that have been developed on the basis of health-related research and established therapeutic techniques. This can include a range of areas, and the examples below are just some instances of how knowledge from this field can be incorporated within library activities.

CST group work, Norwich Prison Library, UK

Cognitive Stimulation Therapy (CST) is a technique that research has found to be suitable for people with mild to moderate dementia. According to a Cochrane review (a systematic review of primary research in health care and health policy prepared and maintained using specific methodologies described in the *Cochrane Handbook*) on the potential benefits of CST for people with dementia, programmes were found to bring cognitive benefits in people with mild to moderate dementia over and above any medication effects. Other outcomes from this approach need more exploration, but improvements in self-reported quality of life and wellbeing were promising (Woods et al., 2012).

Group CST treatment involves 14 or more sessions of themed activities, which typically run twice weekly. The initial sessions may be followed by longer-term 'Maintenance CST'. Sessions aim to actively stimulate and engage people with dementia, whilst offering an opportunity to share experiences and talk with other people with the condition in a relaxed and supportive environment. This can help to build self-esteem, so participants feel better about themselves and more confident to join in conversations and activities. Sessions follow the same structure, usually starting with a warm-up activity, a song and sharing a 'reality orientation board', which has information about the group and details including date, time, place and weather. Members give their group a name and sessions cover a range of activities to stimulate thinking, memory and connection with others, such as discussing current news stories; listening to music or singing; playing word games; or doing a practical activity such as following a recipe (Comas-Herrera and Knapp, 2016).

There are few statistics on the number of people in prisons who have dementia. There can be difficulties in recognising dementia in prison populations owing to a lack of relevant training for staff and the high incidence of concurrent mental health conditions. The extremely regimented routine in place may also serve to mask early symptoms. However, it is estimated that 5% of UK prisoners over 55 may be affected (BACP, 2019). Older prisoners are the fastest growing group in the prison population. The number of prisoners aged 60 or over in England and Wales increased by 243% between 2002 and 2020 (House of Commons Justice Committee, 2020). The rate of suspected dementia and mild cognitive impairment has been estimated as approximately two times higher among prisoners aged 60 to 69 years and four times higher among those aged 70 and over, compared to the same age groups living in the community (Forsyth et al., 2020). Similarly, in the US, the Census Bureau projects that by 2030, people over the age of 55 will account for almost one-third of all incarcerated people and, if researchers' estimates are correct, between 70,000 to 211,000 of the elderly prison population will have dementia (Lopez, 2020).

As Gemma Williams and Judith Farmer (2016) describe, the CST programme at Norwich Prison Library in the UK was devised as a collaboration between the library and a local dementia charity. The main theme of the group changes each week, but might involve having a discussion, playing a game of skittles, doing a quiz, guessing a mystery object or singing. The group has a name and a song chosen by participants. Singing the song at the start of the session is typically followed by brief seated ball games and a 'round robin' group exercise, when each person is invited to share how they are. Interestingly, the team at Norwich Prison Library decided to make some adaptations to the standard format of a CST session – making the approach more person-centred. They found that participants were unresponsive to discussions about the date, time and season, but responded enthusiastically to the team's interest in their world. They therefore swapped the 'orientation in place and time' section of the standard CST session for a slot called 'How has the week been for you?'. The team made further changes when they realised that some themes in the original guide did not engage participants because of the constraints of the prison setting. For example, there was little interest in financial matters and participants were not keen to talk about occupations and family life other than referring to shared childhood experiences (Williams and Farmer, 2016).

Whilst some of the challenges faced in running a CST group in a prison library are similar to those that might be expected elsewhere, such as in a public library, there are also considerations that are unique to the setting. Williams and Farmer (2016) describe how new participants might not be used to talking in a group and, in particular, not used to being offered a choice within the prison environment. The team therefore introduced stress-free options to encourage the decision-making process, such as asking participants which type of hot drink they would like. Everyone in the group, including facilitators, is offered a name badge with their first name clearly visible. At other times, prisoners are routinely addressed only by their title and surname. In the group, the focus is on listening to each other in a supportive and respectful way. The team found that participants have few other opportunities to talk about themselves, often saying they have no other opportunity to be listened to.

At the end of each session, facilitators carry out a review using a simple summary of what worked well and what they might want to change next time. The team undertake Dementia Care Mapping (DCM) (University of Bradford, 2022), a technique that allows them to recognise mood and engagement in each participant and to make the post-group review more structured. The team observed how participants have become more supportive and tolerant of each other, with friendships being strengthened by their shared experiences. Prison staff also reported that participants enjoyed the group and it resulted in increased socialising in communal areas and less withdrawal. Participants started to take noticeably more pride in their appearance, improving personal hygiene and smartening themselves up for the group (Williams and Farmer, 2016).

Table 5.1 shows how the outcomes of the CST sessions at Norwich Prison Library, as reported in Williams and Farmer (2016), can be mapped onto Tom Kitwood's model, described in Chapter 1.

Table 5.1 *Outcomes of CST at Norwich Prison Library mapped onto Kitwood's model*

Attachment	Participants become more supportive and tolerant of each other and friendships are strengthened.
Comfort	The use of first names within the group.
Inclusion	Everyone is encouraged to share their experiences in the group. Participants take part in increased socialising in communal areas and are less withdrawn.
Identity	It is one of the few times when participants are encouraged to share aspects of their lives and how their week has been. Participants smarten themselves up for the group.
Occupation	Participants take part in a variety of activities tailored to their interests and situation. They are offered a choice and encouraged to make decisions.

Distraction therapy collection, Walsall NHS Trust Library, UK

Whilst in some settings, library staff deliver activities for people with dementia directly, in other cases, the role of library staff is focused on the development of collections that allow others to deliver therapeutic activities. The distraction therapy collection at Walsall Healthcare NHS Trust in the UK is an example of the latter. Distraction therapy can be used in a variety of situations, in particular to help manage pain or stressful situations.

The distraction therapy collection includes a range of specialist equipment and was developed as a collaboration between the hospital's Older Adults Mental Health Team, Dementia Support Team and Library and Knowledge Services. Healthcare professionals within the Trust use the equipment to distract and stimulate patients with dementia. They have found this can help to prevent falls and improve sleeping patterns, as well as providing a less stressful experience in hospital for people with dementia. The collection includes computer monitors and tablets with pre-loaded software that can be used to help families and healthcare staff engage patients by providing distraction and stimulation. The software is designed to help with hand-eye co-ordination, promote social interaction, stimulate conversation and distract patients who are agitated. It includes a reminiscence area with music, poetry, radio shows, television clips and feature films, plus an activities area with sing-a-longs, painting, quizzes, jigsaws, armchair exercises and games – including coconut shy, whack-a-mole, shooting gallery and penalty kicks. Other items in the distraction therapy collection include CDs and DVDs (with players); radios; Nintendo DS and games; photo albums (for example, old photos of Walsall); and a 'namaste collection', which includes a motion lamp, beauty case and selection of disposable items such as flannels, toiletries and perfume (Walsall Healthcare NHS Trust, 2019). All the distraction therapy equipment is labelled and added to the library catalogue so items can be tracked. The library team were trained to use the specialist equipment by a dementia support worker. A web page was created to promote the collection and to enable online booking. The library team promote the collection, explain the borrowing procedures to ward managers and carry out regular ward visits to monitor the process.

Liz Askew, Information and Knowledge Specialist at Walsall Healthcare NHS Trust, describes the process of setting up the collection and loaning items:

> Initially, it was about managing the existing collection, doing a stock check and asking, 'What have we got? What bits need replacing?'. And as time went on and we built up a relationship with the mental health and dementia teams, it was more about identifying gaps in provision. We've got a dementia café, for instance, so we needed to get a flask for tea as part of the collection. With the distraction therapy collection, rather than issue it to one person, we invented a ward library card and we also set out a disclaimer to say, 'If you loan the equipment, you've got to look after it, and if anything gets broken, you have to pay for it [from the ward budget]'. So, it was like a loan agreement just to stop things going missing. It's hard to lose the monitors because they're big, so those were given an eight-week loan, but we do ward walks and we'll check equipment is still there and complete.
>
> (L. Askew, conversation with author, 6 December 2021)

Quiet hours

In recent years many supermarkets, as well as other businesses such as gyms, have introduced 'quiet hours' to improve accessibility for people with autism and other conditions. Typically, during this time, a supermarket does not have music or loudspeaker announcements; checkout bleeps are quieter; and staff avoid moving crates of stock around as much as possible. Whilst quiet hours have usually been introduced to make shopping easier for people with autism, they may also be helpful for people with anxiety or other mental health conditions – and of course some people with dementia.

Some libraries have also introduced quiet, or sensory-friendly, hours. For example, Kingsfold Public Library in Lancashire in the UK advertises a quiet hour when customers are asked to mute mobile phones and other devices (Lancashire County Council, 2022). Other libraries have taken this idea further. For instance, several libraries in South Taranaki in New Zealand have weekly sensory hours when artificial lights are dimmed, computers turned off and noisy activities suspended. The hour is aimed at children and adults who may experience difficulties using a large, busy place with lots of noise, lights and people. Although the library staff have not purposely designed the hour for people living with dementia, anyone is welcome to come at this time if they feel the environment will benefit them (A. L. Vonk, e-mail to author, 18 November 2021). Public libraries in Manchester in the UK operate an Age Friendly Hour on one morning per week. This is advertised as a quieter time for older people to pick up library books, read the newspaper or chat with library staff, with free hot drinks and biscuits. Sometimes special activities such as crafts or music are scheduled as part of the Age Friendly Hour (MancLibraries Blog, 2022).

If you are considering introducing a quiet hour in your library, it is worth bearing in mind that, whilst it can have benefits, certain features that are commonly part of this approach, particularly dimmed lighting, may not always be helpful changes for people with dementia. In a larger library, it may be worth experimenting with slightly different sensory environments in different sections of the library to cater for people with differing needs and preferences.

Doll therapy

Some people, particularly in the later stages of dementia, may be soothed and comforted by holding a doll or soft toy animal. These types of toys have been found to bring feelings of relaxation and pleasure to some people with dementia. It is theorised that holding a doll or toy animal may remind people of a time earlier in their life when they had a young child or a pet. The toys can also be a means for carers to make a connection with someone with dementia, by asking them questions or making observations about the doll or animal (Dementia UK, 2020).

Some libraries, such as Bedford Free Public Library (2022) in Massachusetts in the US, loan toy pets and dolls for people with dementia. This can be useful for carers and people with dementia to try out the resources to see whether it is an approach that is likely to work for them. However, it is possible that someone with dementia may become highly attached to the doll or toy animal, so it may be worth having supplier information available for carers who wish to purchase an identical one for someone who responds well. It is also a good idea to provide guidance on the use of doll therapy for people borrowing toy dolls or animals (for example, Dementia UK, 2020) to help them understand how to use the approach effectively and to emphasise the importance of allowing the person with dementia to make their own decisions about if, and how, they interact with the toy.

Carers' groups

Finally, it is worth noting that some libraries run groups offering support to carers. This might be groups explicitly for people caring for someone with dementia, but often includes carers in a variety of situations. Whilst some carers' groups primarily have a social role, often combined with information provision, others offer more therapeutic interventions. For example, Dallas Public Library (2018) in Texas in the US promotes a stressbusting course for caregivers of people with dementia covering stress management techniques, relaxation and coping strategies.

Activities supporting social connections

Whilst some library activities, such as those described above, are based on clinical research and therapies developed within the medical or healthcare sector, others are focused on the value of social interaction. As with many areas of dementia research, the relationship between social interaction and dementia is complex and uncertain. For instance, some studies report that having larger social networks protects against cognitive decline in older adults, whilst others suggest, conversely, that declining cognition and function cause a person's social network to decrease in size (Casey, 2019).

Although there is currently insufficient evidence to link social activity to a reduction in the risk of cognitive decline, or to dementia specifically, social participation and support have been shown to be strongly connected to good health and wellbeing throughout life (WHO, 2019). Furthermore, much of the person-centred approach to dementia care described in Chapter 1 is predicated on the importance of social contact: ensuring people feel included, valued and comforted from being around others. Many libraries already offer social activities for people with dementia and carers. Sometimes this is as part of a broader offer open to a general audience, but in many cases libraries also provide opportunities for social connection for people with dementia specifically. The section below describes a number of social activities and interventions offered in libraries that are aimed at, or accessible to, people with dementia.

Memory cafés

Memory cafés, or dementia cafés, are probably the most widely offered activity for people with dementia and their carers in libraries. A memory café provides a space where people with dementia can go for a cup of tea and a chat with others in a similar position. A memory café can also provide advice and information for those caring for someone with dementia. Memory cafés are intended to be safe, engaging and welcoming meeting spaces. Individual cafés may have a particular focus: some are activity-based or support reminiscence, whilst others focus on education, for example, inviting speakers on different aspects of dementia and sometimes broader topics too. In other cases, memory cafés simply facilitate informal conversations to create new friendships.

Whilst the idea of bringing people together in this type of informal social gathering may sound straightforward, there are issues to consider. Individuals can have different needs and preferences in terms of the size of the group, frequency of meeting, activities offered and so forth. There is no single 'right' type of memory café and it is worth considering how any library-based provision complements other social activities available in the locality.

Another factor to consider is how dementia can affect a person's language and communication skills. For example, as dementia progresses, some people may find it increasingly difficult to communicate in a second language, even if they spoke the language fluently previously. In some areas, therefore, libraries run memory cafés in different languages to cater for the needs of local communities. For example, in the US, libraries often run memory cafés for Spanish speakers. However, there is undoubtedly a need for more memory cafés, as well as other activities, for people with dementia who do not speak the dominant language of the region where they live as their mother tongue.

Let's Talk Dementia Social Group, Kent Libraries, UK
Lynsey Ilett, Customer Services Development Librarian at Folkestone & Hythe District in Kent in the UK, describes a successful memory café-style social group:

Our Let's Talk Dementia project started when we were trying to replicate a reading session I had visited at Canterbury Library. However, I was aware that, at the time, we were lacking an information point in the town. We are lucky to have a very active and well organised Hythe Dementia Forum, run voluntarily by passionate members of the local community. After meeting with a member of the Dementia Forum, we decided that a weekly open session with tea and coffee and information on dementia services would be a good start.

We imagined that the attendees would drift in; have a drink and a chat; take their information; and go off again. From the very start, however, the attendees would stay for the whole session and not only take our information, but would chat to each other and share experiences, and ultimately offer an understanding ear.

The group welcomes anyone interested in, or impacted by, dementia. We have had people with advanced dementia come along with their partners. As we are not trained carers, we had to have a robust plan in place to ensure we are able to manage all situations that may arise. This also means that if someone does come along with advanced dementia, they would need to be accompanied.

We schedule activities, such as memory games, crafts and guest speakers. The Dementia Forum supplies the funds for the hot drinks and other expenditure for activities through regular community fundraisers. It is a delight to say that over the past four years, the group members have become very close friends.

(L. Ilett, e-mail to author, 10 January 2022)

Reminiscence activities

Reminiscence sessions, in which participants share life experiences, memories and stories from the past, are another activity for people with dementia commonly offered in libraries, particularly those with a local history service or archive attached. Some authors describe reminiscence as a therapy. However, I have chosen to discuss it as a social intervention, rather than as a health-related approach, because research evidence on the potential therapeutic benefits of reminiscence activities is inconsistent and can differ considerably across different settings (for example, in care homes or community settings) and approaches (for example, group or individual sessions) (Woods et al., 2018). Furthermore, as reminiscence activities within libraries are mostly delivered as a group activity, it makes sense to focus on the potential social benefits of the activity.

Typically, a person with dementia is often better able to recall events from many years ago than recent memories. Reminiscence draws on this strength; it can give people with dementia a sense of competence and confidence through emphasising a skill they still retain. When a person shares something about their past and another person shows interest or enjoyment, it can be an opportunity for that person to feel that they are the one who is giving something to others, rather than being the one who is always having to have things done for them (SCIE, 2020c). However, it is important to bear in mind that talking about the past can bring up a variety of feelings. Whilst these can often be happy memories and good feelings, reminiscence can sometimes provoke painful memories.

'Do you remember when . . .?' is the question many people might associate with reminiscing. However, it is probably not the best starting point for a person with memory problems. Plain, factual questions (for example, 'How many brothers and sisters did you have?', 'Where were you born?', 'Where did you got to school?') may seem simple but can sometimes be challenging and stressful for people with dementia who may worry they will get the answer wrong or be embarrassed about not being able to remember. An alternative starting point might be to share a memory yourself as a way of leading into asking a question more gently. This can help to give someone clues about the sorts of things they might talk about and may help them to relax and recall their memories more easily, with less fear of mixing things up or forgetting. Alternatively, asking a question that prompts a more imaginative response may help people who are struggling to remember facts to become involved in the discussion in a less pressured way (for example, 'What do you think might be happening in this photo?' or 'Which photo/object do you like best?'). Also, be prepared for responses you may not have anticipated. For example, someone may not respond to a picture of a VE Day party by remembering their experiences on VE Day but might instead remember having a dress similar to one that someone in the photograph is wearing.

Stockton Local History Group, Stockton Reference Library, UK

A local history group for older people and people living with dementia is held every month at Stockton Reference Library in Stockton-on-Tees. The group typically has around eight participants and includes people with dementia who come on their own and those who attend with a carer.

Karen Morris, Health and Wellbeing Librarian at Stockton-on-Tees Borough Council, describes how the group was established and what a typical session looks like:

> I was working with a lovely gentleman who has the most amazing knowledge of local history, but he was telling me that because he has dementia, he was starting to struggle finding pictures using our computers; he kept pressing on the wrong button and losing everything. He was really sad about the fact that he was losing his abilities to use the computer. So I thought, 'I'm sure we can have a structured local history group that is specifically for people who have problems with their cognitive ability, whether it's through dementia or just old age, and they struggle to keep up with technology'.
>
> We host a site called Picture Stockton (https://picturestocktonarchive.com), which is a local history site, and we decided that we would use our photos from there in the group. We would purchase iPads and download photos. Then we would have a group who would meet and swipe through the pictures and chat about whatever they want.

There's no navigation, there's no research for group members to do; we do the legwork, put the photos on the iPads and see what happens. We usually load about 30 pictures, but we never get through 30 pictures in a session; we usually end up having to do half the next time around. We used to have it themed, but now the group just want random photos. They love to be able to sit and talk, and obviously little memories come out as well. They love looking at photos trying to guess what it is and where it is and chat; they just come alive. There's no pressure on them. They just turn up, look at the photos and chat away about whatever they want to chat away about. It works wonderfully.

We all have individual iPads and the reference librarian loads them with the same photos, so everybody swipes along at the same time. We have the picture first and then we have the picture with information about it. They've all got used to swiping. There's no clicking buttons, no navigation. It's very, very simple. If the iPad times out, we have to help them with that. But they're all very good at swiping backwards and forwards and stretching the images to have a closer look. That's the good thing about the tablet: they can stretch the image. But it does mean your photos have to be reasonably good quality, because if they're too grainy, they don't stretch.

We have to facilitate the group carefully. Sometimes people can sort of sit back and drift away and not engage. But as soon as you target them and ask them an open question, that's it: once they start talking, the floodgates just open and they're off. And the rest of the group are really supportive of that because obviously they all understand dementia, so they encourage them to keep talking and ask them questions and they get involved with their own memories.

We make a bookmark with all the meeting dates for the coming year. If we don't see anyone for a few months, we give them a ring to see if there's any reason why: maybe they've just forgotten about it or they've lost confidence.

I would say keep the numbers small to make sure every person is able to be supported. We have two members of staff to eight people, but we also have two carers accompanying two of the people with dementia as well. But don't overwhelm the group because too many members of staff versus participants can be overwhelming in itself. Also, always ask the group members what they want to do and how they want to do it. If they're not enjoying something, you can change it to make it better for them.

(K. Morris, conversation with author, 22 November 2021)

Sporting Memories Clubs

Whilst some reminiscence groups, such as the Stockton Local History Group, focus on a local area, others bring together people who share a common interest. For instance, a number of libraries run Sporting Memories Clubs, sometimes in collaboration with a local sports team. Sporting Memories Clubs are for anyone over the age of 50 who enjoys talking about and remembering sport. Some members are living with dementia, others have low mood or are isolated, but many simply enjoy the opportunity to meet other people. There are both online and community-based clubs attended by fans, former players and family members. Sessions often start with a club song. Sporting Memories produces *Sporting Pink,* a publication with articles and features about historical sporting events, which is often used as a starting point for the week's conversations. Other activities include quizzes and competitions; talking about items of sporting memorabilia; and gentle exercises or physical games (Sporting Memories, n.d.).

Cognitive care kits

This section has focused on social activities that take place within libraries, but it is also important to reflect on the types of resources libraries might provide to encourage social engagement and connection between a person with dementia and a carer, or other friends and family, in their own home or elsewhere. An example is cognitive care kits, which are available for loan in a number of libraries. Cognitive care kits can be designed to support a variety of skills such as communication, hand-eye co-ordination, fine motor skills and attention. Kits typically contain an assortment of activities, games and worksheets that encourage social engagement and participation in daily activities.

The exact content can vary, but the kits available at Vestavia Hills Library in the Forest in Alabama in the US give an idea of the types of materials included. This library loans kits to help support the skills and abilities of people living with early-, mid- and late-stage dementia. The kits have been designed based on recommendations from the Alzheimer's Association, the Dementia Society of America, plus Fit Minds and Relish Dementia Activities, companies that offer specialised activity products for people with dementia. Like most libraries that offer cognitive care kits, Vestavia Hills has a short video describing the kits and giving advice on their use. The early- to mid-stage kit includes a 'match up the sayings' game; a conversation game with picture and conversation prompt cards; a book with large print, short, easy to follow paragraphs and plenty of illustrations designed to prompt reminiscence; large print wordsearches (with no backwards or diagonal words); and colouring sheets (Vestavia Hills Library in the Forest, 2022).

Akron-Summit County Public Library in Ohio in the US has taken a slightly different approach. Working with the Ohio Council for Cognitive Health and other partners, the library has developed a series of memory kits focused on everyday work, leisure or domestic activities, such as gardening, office work and the kitchen. The 'working with tools' memory kit, for instance, includes items such as wood pieces and sandpaper, screws to sort, and locks and keys, as well as a book about woodworking and matching photo and label cards. Kits also include basic information about dementia, tips for carers, guidance for each activity and a list of community resources related to dementia (Akron-Summit County Public Library, 2022).

Arts-related activities

Arts-related activities are the third category of intervention that libraries commonly offer for people with dementia and their carers. Arts-related schemes offered in libraries might include a wide range of activities, including singing or music; drawing or colouring; storytelling; film screenings and concerts; and dance and movement. It is not possible to cover all areas in this book, so the section below focuses on music, theatre and film, and storytelling and creative writing. This section concludes with case studies illustrating how people with dementia might contribute to cultural institutions by supporting collection development in libraries.

Some arts-related activities can be thought of as an extension of libraries' core activities; for example, around reading and literacy, or supporting customers in finding and curating various types of resources, such as music. In some cases the arts activities offered may draw on the particular skills or background of individual staff members. However, this is also an area where partnership working can play an important role as libraries collaborate with artists and arts organisations to deliver services.

It is now widely accepted that participative arts are important for enriching the lives of people with dementia (APPG on Arts, Health and Wellbeing, 2017). Creative expression through artistic activities such as painting or music has been shown to be an important way for people with dementia to express and access emotions despite changes in their cognitive abilities (for example, McLean, 2011; Zeilig et al., 2014). In particular, it has been suggested that creative activities can be helpful to address behavioural and emotional changes in dementia, such as reducing agitation (for example, Cowl and Gaugler, 2014; Lin et al., 2011).

Music

Research is increasingly demonstrating the positive effects of music for people with dementia. This is an art form where both research and practice in working with people with dementia is particularly strong (Music for Dementia, n.d.). Music can trigger emotions, feelings and memories in people, particularly when there is a personal connection to their past experiences. Interacting with music can be 'passive', such as listening to recorded or live music, or 'active', when people are involved in making music through playing an instrument or singing. The case studies below include examples of how libraries can support both types of activity.

Playlist creation

Libraries often support musical playlist creation for people with dementia. A number of libraries across the UK, for instance, have signed up to become Playlist for Life Help Points. Playlist for Life is a music and dementia charity that supports people with dementia to have a unique, personal playlist that those who care for them know how to use. A 'Playlist for Life' is made up of music with strong memories or emotions attached (Playlist for Life, 2019). Using technology can be one of the biggest challenges faced by people when making a playlist, so libraries can help by providing internet access and trained volunteers to support people. Library staff or volunteers help carers, or people with dementia themselves, to create a playlist to help to evoke memories, prompt conversations and strengthen relationships. Furthermore, through access to music libraries such as Freegal (www.freegalmusic.com/home), many libraries have a cheap and easy way for users to access music.

One example is the AK Bell Library in Perth, Scotland, which hosts a Playlist for Life Information Hub each month run by volunteers. The volunteers promote Playlist for Life to the general public and particularly to carers of people with dementia. They provide information about Playlist for Life, such as a list of music through the decades that might encourage positive and significant memories for the people with dementia; discuss and demonstrate the different devices that can be used for Playlist for Life (iPad, MP3 player, etc.); and assist carers and the general public to download music to create their playlist (Culture Perth & Kinross, 2016).

Singing groups

Several libraries offer singing groups for people with dementia, often in partnership with local musicians or singers. As might be expected, it has been difficult to keep singing groups going during the COVID-19 pandemic and Chapter 6 includes an example of an online singing group that was able to continue throughout Covid lockdowns. Heather Rodenhurst, Team Librarian from Shropshire Libraries in the UK, describes her experiences of trying to restart a face-to-face group following the easing of COVID-19 restrictions.

> Even before the pandemic, there were only three Singing for the Brain groups [an intervention based on group singing activities developed by the UK Alzheimer's Society for people with dementia and their carers] happening in Shropshire; three of the main towns had sessions, but nowhere else. So, there definitely is a gap. I've been a singer all my life, so I thought, 'This is something we could do in libraries'.
>
> It's so lovely to have that experience where you see people who were quite badly affected by dementia suddenly able to join in. I notice in group settings,

where there are organised activities going on, it might often be that the carer with the person with dementia is getting a great deal out of the conversation or exchange of information. The person with dementia can also be participating and getting something out of it, but there are always those who are not able to participate fully; they're not following the conversation and understanding what's been put in front of them. But if you start singing a song that they know, there's that magic thing; the lyrics are still there in their heads and they're singing along with everybody else. And for that short time, everybody's on the same footing, just enjoying this lift in spirit. And you also know that even if the singing only lasts five minutes, that uplift will stay with the person with dementia for a while afterwards, so that's great for them. It's great for the carer too.

The group's not only open to people with dementia; there are older people on their own and they really get a lift out of singing with others. I think there's a real need there. It's been slower to get going after the pandemic than I thought it would be. I think that there are still people who are feeling too vulnerable to be out and about, or they've just lost that confidence and have got used to a more kind of secluded, restricted routine at home.

I think you've got to feel quite comfortable because I don't bring an instrument with me; it's just acapella. I'm happy to run it with six or eight people, but I think less than that would mean it's less comfortable for people to sing. I have a folder of lyrics and people pick what they want to sing. I became aware that you don't want to enforce your ideas of what a song for somebody with dementia should be because you really have no idea. We sing the 'White Cliffs of Dover', but we also sing the Beatles, Elvis Presley, Roger Whittaker . . . It's really hard to find up-to-date song books for people to use though. Some are quite dated and the songs are for older generations really, rather than the people we're seeing with dementia in the library.

One woman was quite emotional because she'd said at the beginning, 'I can't sing'. And she's got a really good voice, so I said, 'How come you think you can't sing?'. And she said, 'I've always been told I can't sing. I was told as a child'. I hear that so much, so on the posters I put, 'Everyone can sing!'. You know, sometimes it's a little out of tune, but it doesn't matter . . .

(H. Rodenhurst, conversation with author, 30 May 2022)

Theatre and film

People with dementia can find it difficult to access mainstream theatre performances or cinema screenings. Dementia-friendly performances and screenings are therefore becoming increasingly common in theatres and cinemas. Libraries that have a space to host screenings or performances often offer these too.

Film screenings

For those libraries with a suitable, accessible space, dementia-friendly film screenings can be a popular activity. An example is Mansfield Central Library in the UK, which offers regular dementia-friendly screenings of classic films and musicals, such as *On Moonlight Bay*, *Funny Face* and *Pillow Talk*. Although these screenings are designed for people with dementia or memory challenges, everyone is welcome and some films are screened during school holidays so families can attend together. Audience members are free to talk, sing and move around during the screening. The film is paused in the middle for an interval. There is also a quiet room nearby for anyone needing a break from the film and volunteers to support anyone who needs help (Inspire, 2022).

Theatre productions

As well as performances and screenings for people with dementia, there are examples of productions about dementia aimed at carers and wider audiences. One is Gaye Poole's play *Connie's Colander*, which toured UK libraries in 2018 and 2019. An evaluation of this tour (Lewis et al., 2019) found that attending the performance helped audiences to learn about dementia and the ways it can affect both people with dementia and their carers. Carers appreciated seeing their experiences represented on stage and gained ideas and coping strategies for living with dementia. There was positive feedback about the fact that the performance took place in libraries; audiences felt the setting was friendly, relaxed, welcoming and accessible. The intimacy of the space meant many people felt more included in the performance than they might be in a larger venue. Library staff also reported that the performance helped them to empathise more with people affected by dementia and better understand the issues they face.

Storytelling and creative writing

Whilst music and performance activities utilise the resources and spaces available in libraries, storytelling and creative writing activities draw more specifically on libraries' expertise in literature and language and can be closely linked to reading activities, such as those described in Chapter 4. As yet, however, the potential of storytelling and creative writing activities for people with dementia in libraries is relatively under-exploited.

Storytelling

Storytelling can be closely linked to some of the types of reading activities described in Chapter 4, such as ways of reading together. However, it is more explicitly focused on oral stories and skills rather than written texts. Some libraries host adult storytelling sessions and often these are aimed at, or designed to be inclusive of, people with dementia. The care home where my dad lived, Belong Crewe, was involved in a project with Bluecoat arts centre in Liverpool. Called Where the Arts Belong, the project involved opportunities for residents, many of whom are living with dementia, to engage with a range of arts activities (Bluecoat, n.d.). This included storytelling activities, such as story bingo and creating a group story based around an image. The latter has similarities to Timeslips activities (www.timeslips.org/resources/creativity-center), which some libraries have used. It involved asking a series of questions about an image, such as 'Who are the people in the picture?', 'Where are they going?', 'What are they doing?', and using the responses to build up a collaborative story based around the image that could then be told, or read back, to the group by the facilitator (Postlethwaite, 2021). This activity by Natalie Ravenscroft at Belong Crewe was developed in partnership with the Bluecoat and was inspired by an original activity by Roger Hill.

Creative writing

Many libraries host creative writing groups and activities, run either by library staff or by external facilitators, and there are a few examples of creative writing groups specifically for people with dementia. However, too often there is a perception that people with dementia will not be able to engage in creative writing. In fact, people in the early stages of dementia may well be able to participate in what we would normally think of as a creative writing group – although they may need more time to complete activities or support, such as someone to scribe or read for them. For people in the later stages of dementia, creative writing is still possible through thinking more broadly about what we mean by writing (just as many of the activities suggested in Chapter 4 are based on a broader idea of what 'reading' involves).

In its most basic definition, writing is 'making marks, letters, words or other symbols on a surface' (McMillan and McNicol, 2019). As part of the Where the Arts Belong project, introduced above, artist Tabitha Moses ran mark making activities with care home residents. Mark making is a technique commonly used by artists to express their feelings or emotions about something they have seen or experienced. 'Marks' are lines, dots, marks, patterns or textures that can be applied by any materials onto a surface. Whilst not what many people might initially consider this as 'writing', mark making can be a way for people with dementia to express and share their emotions and responses. In the mark making activity for care home residents, participants were encouraged to make marks using pastels on paper in response to their reactions to pieces of instrumental music that were played to the group. This meant that participants were encouraged to produce their own artistic response to each piece of music, but there was no pressure on them to either produce an accomplished drawing or to write using letters and words.

Another possibility for creative writing is to make use of resources such as the MakeWrite app (https://blogs.city.ac.uk/inca/makewrite). This was designed for people with the language disorder aphasia but can be suitable for people with dementia more broadly. The app allows you to use existing texts to produce your own new piece of creative writing in four stages: choose a source text, erase text to leave words you want to use, arrange the words into a new text and share your creation. It is a similar idea to cut-up ('found') poetry, a simple version of which can be used as a non-digital alternative. For a brief description of found poetry techniques, see https://poetryteatime.com/blog/found-poetry.

As with storytelling activities, co-authorship can be an effective way to approach creative writing for people with dementia; it means there is less pressure on individuals and it can make writing a more collaborative, social process. An example of how this can work in practice comes from an Arts Council England-funded project where professional artists and a peer support group for people with dementia worked together over a series of workshops to create a comic about living with the condition (McNicol and Leamy, 2020). Activities that took place in the workshops included discussing the impact of living with dementia on participants' daily lives; deciding on key messages for the comic; providing feedback on character design and constructing character biographies; deciding on a title for the comic; plotting potential storylines; and commenting on a series of progressively more developed drafts of the comic sketched by the artist. Through this process, group members acted as co-authors, making a direct contribution to the creation of a published comic. Detailed guidance on this approach is available at www.sarahmcnicol.co.uk/theres-no-bus-map-for-dementia.

Collection development

Another way that people with dementia can be involved in artistic and cultural activities is through contributing to the development of a library collection. A number of libraries seek advice and suggestions from people with dementia and carers when purchasing resources about, or to support people living with, the condition. However, people with dementia can also work with library staff to develop aspects of the collection in more creative ways. As the case studies below illustrate, this can bring benefits for both the library service and people with dementia.

Sefton's Lost Voices, Sefton Library Service, UK
Sefton's Lost Voices project gives people in the early stages of memory loss the chance to record their oral histories (Sefton Council, 2022). The interviewee receives a copy of the recording, which they can share with family and friends, and in some cases a copy is also retained by the local history archive.

Lesley Davies, Senior Development Manager at Sefton Library Services in the UK, describes how the project works:

> The main thrust of Lost Voices is to record people who are in the early stages of dementia. We worked with the North West Sound Archive who gave some volunteers, myself and a couple of colleagues some training on interview techniques for archives. So we were able to train our first cohort of volunteers and ever since then, myself and a couple of colleagues have done the training for the volunteers. We manage the service; we take the bookings; we deal with the care homes; and we'd go out and speak to the care homes before volunteers went out. But the volunteers do the recording. So it's a volunteer-run service led by the library.
>
> We thought we'd be absolutely inundated with people who wanted to record their memories, but very few people came forward initially. We found it's no good just setting it up and expecting people to come to you. Because when you've got a diagnosis of dementia, the last thing you're thinking about is recording your memories really. So there is some work to do to get people in. We were initially working with the Alzheimer's Society, then we went to memory clinics and then we started to go to care homes as well. We would go into a care home on a certain afternoon for a number of weeks. I would say it's 60–65% care homes, around 30% community, although that includes community groups, such as the local older people's partnership as well. So the proportion of people coming forward themselves to be interviewed, I would say it's probably about 10%.
>
> Before the interview, we send out a little form asking their name, their age and if they have any health issues that we should be aware of, just so the volunteer is not going in blind. And then we ask them, 'Is there a particular area of their life that they'd like to talk about?'. Sometimes it's their career; sometimes it's their school; sometimes it's their home life. We ask some basic questions to start with, so we've got some context for the recording, but we try and back off as much as possible and just let them talk. We have some prompt questions if they get stuck. The recordings usually last about 20 minutes to half an hour. We burn the recording to a CD for the person and their family, and if relevant we would do a recording for our archive. For example, we interviewed someone who worked at the first brain injury centre, which is nearby. So we've had some really, really interesting stories about its history that we'd never know about otherwise. We broadcast the ones that were really interesting in a 12-month series through our social media channels.
>
> We've had quite a few family members come back and say, 'We've learned things that we didn't know'. For families, it can mean a great deal that they can share their grandparents' history and equally it then allows the grandchildren to be able to

converse with grandparents who sometimes you haven't got that connection with if you don't know an awful lot about their life. It's lovely to be able to have the recording, to able to say, 'I was listening to your tape and you're talking about what you did . . .'. So we've heard from children and grandchildren who've been able to reconnect.

Care homes have used the CDs at their reminiscence sessions as well. Some of the homes started to say, 'We've played this person's recording and we've all started to discuss it', because a few people were at the same school or worked in the same place. It's started conversations within the group and they know a lot more about the person than perhaps they had done previously.

We had to pause the project during Covid of course, but going forward we're looking at whether we can use mobile phones or tablets as a recording device rather than dictaphones, because then we can edit it a little bit easier. We're also looking at whether CDs are appropriate to send out to people anymore because that's old technology really. We might ask people if they would like a CD or an MP3 file. And the other thing we're looking at is trying to make more of a pack for somebody. We've taken photographs of the person that we've recorded so that we can keep that with our copy. Sometimes they would have an old photograph too, so we could have a photograph of them young and old. But now we're wondering, 'Is there a way to add a bit more information?'. So if they're talking about school, for example, have we got a photograph in our archive of the school that we can provide to the person? Or is there a newspaper article? We're going to try that, but it's a bit of trial and error at the moment to see how that works.

(L. Davies, conversation with author, 1 April 2022)

Reminiscence collection, Stockton-on-Tees Libraries, UK
Karen Morris, Health and Wellbeing Librarian at Stockton-on-Tees Borough Council, describes a spin-off project involving a member of the Stockton Local History Group (described above). This extended the group's involvement from looking at and talking about existing photographs to helping to add to the library collection.

We did a spin-off project with one of the gentlemen from the Local History Group. We'd pick pictures from the suburb of Stockton where the man lives from our photo database, Picture Stockton, and then we went back and re-photographed them as near as we could. We even had to go into an estate agent to ask if we could take a photo from the flat upstairs to try to recreate those pictures. It was really good and we've added that to our reminiscence collection. We also made it into a playlist for the immersive experience room [see Chapter 3] so you feel like you're within the pictures. It's my aim to continue that project in the future because I just think people get so much from it. That feeling of worth and that feeling of contributing is massive – the feeling of being useful again.

(K. Morris, conversation with author, 22 November 2021)

Conclusions

The examples in this chapter illustrate just some of the types of activities that libraries might offer for people with dementia and their carers. As the case studies demonstrate, a wide range of activities is possible and these will vary depending on the needs of customers, other initiatives available in the local area and the organisations libraries choose to partner with. Most of the activities described in this chapter were designed to take place, primarily, face-to-face. However, in recent years, and since the COVID-19 pandemic, increasing attention has been paid to the potential use of online and other digital technologies in the provision of activities and services for people with dementia and their carers. Chapter 6 explores some ways in which libraries have adapted their services for people with dementia to make greater use of online and digital technologies.

6
Digital and Online Provision

It's been such a lifeline to some incredibly vulnerable people who struggle to leave home to take part in groups and activities.
(Caroline Varney-Bowers, Community Librarian, Norfolk Library and Information Service, UK)

This chapter explores the use of technology in support of activities for people with dementia and their carers. This can take a variety of forms: some activities involving technology take place within the library, but technology can also make activities and services more accessible for people who might not be able to visit a library easily. The COVID-19 pandemic has accelerated the use of technology in many fields, including library services, and has prompted libraries to pilot more ambitious online activities for people with dementia as it became impossible to run face-to-face activities. Restrictions imposed due to COVID-19, and the understandable reluctance of some older and more vulnerable people to attend in-person activities even when restrictions had been lifted, mean that many library services have placed a stronger focus on delivering online activities than was previously the case. This chapter therefore reflects on some of these Covid-related initiatives, the challenges faced and how they might inform the development of dementia-inclusive online activities on a long-term basis.

Delivering online activities for people with dementia can be extremely challenging for practical reasons: people may lack digital skills or have limited confidence using new technology. There can also be additional challenges in engaging and communicating with people with dementia via a screen where it can be more difficult to convey body language and establish eye contact. Nevertheless, many activities have met with some success.

This chapter starts with a brief overview of some of the considerations around digital and online provision for people with dementia. It then describes a number of online activities offered via libraries, as well as other ways in which technology is being used by libraries to support activities for people with dementia. The chapter concludes by outlining some of the considerations around online provision for those caring for someone with dementia. The focus in this chapter is on library services and activities. Examples of how technology can be incorporated into library design, for instance through the creation of sensory spaces, are discussed in Chapter 3.

Online activity provision for people with dementia

There is relatively little research into the ways in which online and digital services and activities can be designed to be inclusive of people with dementia. Research that does exist is mostly around discrete projects working with a small group of people, rather than mainstream services. However, this has started to change since the beginning of the COVID-19 pandemic in 2020 when the use of video conferencing platforms, such as Zoom and Teams, became increasingly common. The following examples of recent research have similarities to some of the types of activities introduced by libraries.

For instance, Sophie Lee and colleagues carried out research into online dementia-inclusive singing groups in Ireland. They found that delivering the sessions online could be more inclusive of people who live remotely, have mobility issues or struggle travelling to in-person sessions. Online provision was also seen to allow flexibility for days when people with dementia are reluctant to leave the house or feel unwell. However, lack of electronic devices and good internet connections excluded a number of participants from the online groups (Lee et al., 2021).

Similarly, Claire Molyneux and colleagues explored the challenges and benefits of online delivery of music therapy sessions in rural Essex in the UK. Their report offers detailed suggestions around the practicalities of online sessions. Whilst Together in Sound, the project their research is based around, provides music therapy, much of the general guidance and recommendations would equally apply to many other types of online activities for people with dementia. They recommend the creation of a simple but detailed document explaining how to join the session and use the software; practice sessions using the software; telephoning participants prior to and during sessions to provide technical guidance and support; and following up with participants after sessions. They also found that replicating the familiar format of the in-person sessions as much as possible was helpful for participants.

As other projects have also reported, online delivery meant the project was able to reach participants who otherwise would not be able to attend sessions in the community. For some participants living with dementia, there was a high degree of engagement with the screen, while for others, it was much harder to engage. There were some couples where the person with dementia chose not to sit in front of the screen but might stay in the same room. It is more difficult to make use of body language, gesture and eye contact online, so communication has to be more explicit. Molyneux et al. (2020) emphasise the importance of facilitators looking at their camera, rather than at the screen, to help participants experience a sense of connectedness, and using big gestures and simple verbal communications to support actions or instructions. Online sessions are easily dominated by verbal communication instead of body movements or facial expressions, which means that it is more difficult to 'hear' from people with dementia who are less verbal. The team at Together in Sound found that having two facilitators made it easier to notice changes in participants' movements or facial expressions that might indicate they wanted to contribute (Molyneux et al., 2020).

Many of the experiences reported in this research reflect those of library staff who ran online activities during the pandemic. The following section outlines some projects that have taken place in libraries or similar cultural organisations and reflects on the lessons learnt from these experiences.

Online intergenerational arts workshops, The National Archives, UK

The UK National Archives, in partnership with Innovations in Dementia Community Interest Company (CIC), ran an intergenerational online outreach project in 2021. Connecting through Collections (The National Archives, n.d.) brought together older women living with dementia and 17- to 21-year-olds to explore history, art and dementia through a series of intergenerational arts workshops in a women-only online space.

Sara Griffiths from The National Archives describes the practicalities of organising this project:

> I was concerned about running a project online initially as we hold such store by meeting people personally, shaking their hands and making eye contact; it is harder to sense how people are getting on or gain that feedback when a workshop is done online. However, the geographic reach of the project was amazing. Also, we found that whereas normally some people would not attend all sessions because illness would prevent their physical attendance, running the project online allowed even those who were poorly on the day to dip in and out, sometimes from their beds. They would not have had the energy to travel so turnout was generally very good.
>
> I would advise people new to working with dementia to look to professionals in that field and work with experienced practitioners. Our partners, Innovations in Dementia, act as gatekeepers; they have the knowledge and experience to help us shape the project to deliver the most effective and appropriate results for our participants. We

arranged training by one of their participants so that we could be aware of some of the important things to keep in mind and our artists undertook this training with us too. We distributed yellow 'I want to speak' cards for people to hold up if they wished to contribute because we recognised that they might not be able to keep things in mind whilst waiting their turn to speak. Raising a card like this allowed them to be heard quickly and as a priority. We planned frequent short breaks to allow people to take comfort breaks and have time away from the screen.

The older women with dementia were unknown to us, but most knew each other and had already become used to working in an online environment. The young people were quite gifted artistically and we had worked with them previously. We did this deliberately as we felt we needed to have some 'knowns'. We were extremely lucky with our participants; the whole project had an air of openness and honesty about it. We had wondered how comfortable the two generations would be with each other, but there was learning on both sides and the bonds made as a result seemed far easier than I expected for an online environment. We considered opening the project to both male and female participants, but I made the decision to keep it women-only as I felt there was a need to provide an open, honest space for women and I felt it would encourage easier familiarisation and comfort, especially amongst the young people.

We spent a lot of time planning the activities and focusing on what was important in terms of outcomes. We set out and agreed our aims and objectives and went through them with the participants as well. One of the major aims was for the participants to have fun and to learn about each other and we felt successful in achieving that.

Working online with artistic activities was a challenge. Both artists have worked with people with dementia for many years. One of the artists was already quite experienced at delivering online and we found that those sessions working with pen and ink provided a meditative experience that the participants enjoyed. Our other artist had to find ways of showing her work – she pre-filmed a video that the participants could replay and also hooked up a separate camera on her workstation to enable people to watch her hands live while doing the collage activity. We did a few pre-runs as our collage artist hadn't used Zoom before. As dementia can affect fine motor skills and vision, collage, which involved having to cut out shapes from a piece of paper, was not something that we would recommend again, although our artist had tried to anticipate this by cutting out many shapes, which were posted to participants beforehand.

Both artists we worked with put a huge amount of thought into the activity that went beyond what we would normally do on a workshop. We sent out archival copies for each workshop as well as a selection of art basics – glue, brushes, scissors, etc. – working on the basis that people might not have these to hand. This created a level playing field and also some excitement and anticipation!

For each project, we usually finish with a sharing activity where people showcase the work they created; talk about the project; and share tea and cake. Obviously, for an online project it wasn't possible to come together so our final envelope included a choice of tea bags and biscuits. People were really excited and amused to open those! It seemed a fitting end.

Even with this planning, not everything went according to plan – sessions overran and our workshop on Suffragettes created so much discussion and interest, we didn't even get around to the art activity. Sometimes you have to let go and go with the flow as long as the project isn't adversely affected. We were more than delighted with the outcome.

(S. Griffiths, e-mail to author, 30 November 2021)

Online singing workshops, Norfolk Library and Information Service, UK

The National Archives' Connecting through Collections initiative was a discrete project. However, Norfolk Library and Information Service took a slightly different approach as they used video conferencing to allow them to continue to deliver a regular session, which had previously taken place face-to-face in the library, during the COVID-19 lockdown in the UK.

Caroline Varney-Bowers, Community Librarian at Norfolk Library and Information Service in the UK, describes how they organised these sessions:

> For many years, I've worked with a local organisation called Come Singing to offer a regular singing session at our central library in Norwich. Come Singing is a voluntary organisation formed with the aim of providing therapeutic singing sessions specifically for people living with dementia and their carers around Norfolk. Before Covid, the group was meeting on a monthly basis with around 45 people attending.
>
> During the pandemic, we stopped meeting in person but found ways to continue. Initially, we moved to filming a session a month to include on our library's YouTube channel. But after hearing from a colleague that she had successfully brought together her reminiscence group on a Teams group call, we decided to try something similar with the singing group.
>
> All that is required is a phone number for each participant. I use Teams to phone the session leader from Come Singing who is at home sat at her piano ready to lead the session. Then, one by one, I phone each participant – up to around seven people at a time. During the group call, we sing together, chat, hear some solo performances, take requests and generally feel connected by singing together. Sometimes there can be a bit of a time delay online, but no one seems to mind.
>
> On occasions when people have been unwell, they have still wanted to take part but chose just to listen in rather than sing as they enjoy the connection. Sometimes the person with dementia and their carer (which is usually their partner) join in together. We also include a volunteer who used to support the in-person group as it is nice for everyone to keep in touch.
>
> It's been such a lifeline to some incredibly vulnerable people who struggle to leave home to take part in groups and activities. We want to continue with the online version in the future as it allows people to take part if they are not well enough to attend the library, and potentially offers it across the whole county rather than in one location.
>
> (C. Varney-Bowers, e-mail to author, 16 November 2021)

Other technologies for people with dementia

In addition to online events and activities, there are other ways in which libraries are making use of technology to support people with dementia. The following are just two examples of ways in which technology might be used to enhance services.

Digital jigsaws

A number of local studies libraries and archives have created online jigsaws of some of their holdings using software such as Jigsaw Explorer (www.jigsawexplorer.com) or Jigsaw Planet (www.jigsawplanet.com). For example, Toronto Public Library in Canada has digital puzzles of items in its special collection. These range in difficulty from 15-piece to 200-piece puzzles and include items such as an image from a 1928 seed catalogue, a 1912 map of Ontario and a jelly advert from the 1930s (Toronto Public Library, 2020). With most jigsaw software, you can alter the number of pieces in the puzzle and either fix the pieces or allow them to rotate to increase or decrease the level of difficulty, depending on the needs and abilities of the individual playing. It is worth bearing in mind that people with dementia may be more likely to need to see a copy of the image they are trying to piece together, so it is worth including instructions explaining how to display this if it does not appear onscreen automatically.

Another factor to consider is that many archive images, for instance old photographs, will be monochrome. These may be more difficult for people with dementia to complete, so it is worth trying to include more colourful images, especially pictures with contrasting colours, bearing in mind that blues, greens and purples may be more difficult for some people with dementia to distinguish from each other.

Magic tables

A 'magic table' projects interactive light games that are specifically designed to promote social interaction and engagement amongst people living with dementia. They can also be used for children or adults with learning disabilities and autism. Light animations are projected onto a table and, as players reach out towards them, the lights respond to their hand and arm movements. Tovertafel (www.tover.care/uk) is one of the most well-known brands of magic table. Tovertafel games have been designed specifically for people with varying stages of dementia and they can be played both individually and in groups. Games include gardening, fishing and popping bubbles. A number of library services have installed a Tovertafel, including Guernsey Libraries in the Channel Islands, which purchased a Tovertafel with funding from Dementia Friendly Guernsey.

Jackie Burgess, Community and Outreach Librarian at Guernsey Libraries, describes their experiences:

> When we saw the Tovertafel demonstrated, we really, really wanted it. We thought it was just a great service for us to reach out to people with dementia. For people that have got dementia and their carers it can be difficult to go to the main library on Guernsey – it's very tricky sometimes to get a parking place –

but we've got four community libraries around the island that are more easily accessible. So we put the Tovertafel in one of our community libraries that has got easy access car parking. Our community library is in a complex with extra care housing, so we thought that there'd be quite a few residents from the extra care housing that would come down and to look at it and use it. In another building on the same site, there is a lovely café. So I thought, 'They can come to us and then go and have a cup of tea and a piece of cake'. We did a few open days and the local press, radio stations and TV stations all came down. And we invited lots of people from the community, people from all the care homes, activity co-ordinators and anyone else that we could think of, and it was a really big success. Everybody that looked at the Tovertafel and used it really seemed to enjoy it.

We have about 16 games and activities for the Tovertafel, but my favourite one is like paintball: these big round paint balls roll onto the table and when you slap them, it makes a painting. Once the painting is finished, it turns round so that everyone around the table can see what it is. There's also an activity with flowers: when you press the table, the flowers grow. When we used that, we gave people real flowers to hold as well, which adds an extra element. There's another game like a jigsaw: you put the pieces in to make a picture of a telephone or some old sports equipment, for example. So that's like reminiscence too and it's nice because you can try and encourage people to start talking.

We started to get groups of people coming into the library from different care homes. We've had a drop-in running ever since we installed the Tovertafel, so people can just drop in and they don't have to book. And then if people would like to have myself or a colleague join them for a more private session, we can set that up as well. I find most people are laughing and enjoying sitting at the table, just being together. Staff from care homes have seen a difference when they've got a resident who hasn't been interested in anything, but then has responded to the Tovertafel.

(J. Burgess, conversation with author, 24 November 2021)

However, whilst the technology itself has been well-received, there have been issues around getting care home residents to the community library to use the Tovertafel. These logistical issues, and potential solutions, are discussed further in Chapter 7.

Online provision for carers

The focus of this chapter so far has been online and digital resources for people with dementia. However, it is also important to consider the ways in which online provision might help to support carers. In many ways, considerations around online provision for carers are similar to those for any customer group, for example access to technology, personal preferences and digital skills and confidence. However, online provision can help to overcome some of the challenges carers often face that can be a barrier to attending activities face-to-face, in particular the need to arrange respite care for the person they are caring for. The flexibility of online provision can be important for carers whose time is often highly limited. It can also be more relaxing to know they remain nearby throughout the session and are able to deal with any emergencies if necessary.

Online Dementia Action Week events, Libraries Unlimited, UK

Libraries Unlimited, the public library service for the county of Devon in the UK, ran a series of events for Dementia Action Week in May 2021. This included sessions aimed at the general public, for example dementia awareness sessions, as well as sessions for carers, such as a Q&A with an Admiral Nurse. (Admiral Nurses are specialist dementia nurses who are supported and developed by Dementia UK: www.dementiauk.org/get-support/what-is-an-admiral-nurse). There were also several sessions targeted towards people with dementia, including a taster session of Singing for Wellbeing for Dementia, craft sessions, cookery and bingo. The experiences of Libraries Unlimited targeting different audiences highlights some of the potential differences between running online activities for carers and for people with dementia.

Charlotte Sumner, Team Leader from Paignton Library, describes some of the challenges the library service experienced, but also the potential benefits and lessons learnt about offering sessions in this way:

> I worked with a small group of people from different libraries across Devon, as well as people like the local Admiral Nurse and an organisation called Home Instead, who run our fraud awareness and dementia awareness courses. The biggest challenge we had is people being able to access the events. In some ways, it makes it more available to everybody if you're online, but then not everybody has internet access or the skills to access things online. We had quite a lot of people saying that they would have come if it was in person. On the other hand, if you're looking after somebody, you can't always get out to go and attend something. If it's online, you can just watch it whilst you're at home with them. So being online could be easier for carers. But for sessions that were more for the individual with dementia themselves, I felt they didn't engage through the screen as well as they probably would to an actual person in front of them.
>
> (C. Sumner, conversation with author, 8 December 2021)

Reading is Caring online workshops, Scottish Book Trust

Scottish Book Trust's Reading is Caring pilot project (described in Chapter 4) offered training sessions for carers via Zoom. These were initially planned to be delivered face-to-face, but due to COVID-19 restrictions most had to take place online. Carers' experiences of these sessions reflect many of the considerations reported by other projects offering online support and activities for carers.

Many carers in this project felt that online sessions made it easier for them to attend the Reading is Caring workshops as they did not have to arrange respite care or travel. This could be particularly important for those in more remote locations. As more people became used to using Zoom during the pandemic, for example to attend online dementia friends groups, some of the technical barriers that might otherwise have existed were reduced. However, despite the availability of extensive written and individual technical support for participants, there were, inevitably, some carers who were reluctant, or unable, to attend online sessions.

The Reading is Caring sessions were delivered to individuals or small groups of up to three people. The workshop facilitator felt that it would be more difficult to deliver to larger groups effectively online and maintain the ability for people to interact in a natural way. However, this meant that peer learning was more limited than would have been the case in slightly larger face-to-face groups. The pilot project evaluation recommended that if online delivery is to be considered an element of the Reading is Caring programme in the long term, it may be worth considering ways in which additional support can be provided to compensate for the lack of direct peer-to-peer support during the sessions, such as a Facebook group or other online community where people can share ideas, suggest texts and so forth (McNicol and Dalton, 2021).

Conclusions

There is a need for more research into online and digital provision for people with dementia. There are potential advantages of online provision, in particular in relation to access for people who may find it difficult to attend face-to-face activities for a variety of reasons, including health, transport, confidence and location. However, from what we know so far, it would seem that the success of online services for people with dementia is highly dependent on context. Anecdotally, I saw this in my experiences with my dad. Whilst he would probably have preferred to see me in person, he was happy to chat to me online and was even quite excited to see me 'on the telly'. However, he was less keen to speak to his GP via a videocall.

Experiences such as those described by The National Archives and Norfolk Library and Information Service in the UK demonstrate that it is possible to run successful online activities for people with dementia. However, this is undoubtedly challenging and requires significant preparation and support. Familiarity, in terms of the activity and the technology used, naturally helps. Working with small groups with whom the facilitators have, or can develop, an ongoing relationship typically makes online communication easier. However, larger online events, open to a wider audience, can present significant challenges for people with dementia that can be more difficult to overcome.

As several of the case study interviewees from this and previous chapters emphasised, partnerships with organisations with expertise in dementia are a key consideration when devising and running activities for people with dementia, whether face-to-face or online. This is important not only in the practical delivery of initiatives, but also to ensure that library staff are aware of the latest developments in thinking about dementia care and can plan the library's role to provide the greatest benefits for people with dementia and their carers. However, partnership working is often complex and Chapter 7 explores issues around collaboration beyond the library in greater detail.

7
Partnership Working

> . . . it's always an uphill challenge to get to the right people.
> (Heather Rodenhurst, Shropshire Libraries, UK, in conversation with author)

Partnership working is a crucial aspect of the provision of library services for people with dementia and their carers. Partner organisations, including care homes, day centres, adult social care, arts organisations, community groups and dementia research organisations, can provide valuable guidance and expertise, as well as practical support and even the development of co-delivered services. This can be achieved through both formal strategic partnerships and more ad hoc collaborations. Conversations with potential partners can help to develop library-based activities, but can also lead to the establishment of outreach services to allow libraries to reach people with dementia and their carers in a range of settings. The case studies in Chapters 4 and 5 included examples of partnerships to deliver both library-based and outreach initiatives, but this chapter looks more explicitly at the mechanisms behind the delivery of these types of services – how partnerships are established and maintained – rather than at the services themselves in detail.

Heather Rodenhurst from Shropshire Libraries in the UK describes the importance of both established and more informal, or developing, partnerships to spread the word about the memory bags service they offer (described in Chapter 4):

> The library service is a member of the Shropshire, Telford and Wrekin Dementia Action Alliance. So that's a really good vehicle for us; when the group meets every other month, I can always give them an update. But a lot of it is also

through word of mouth. A local care home had heard about the project and wanted to donate a small sum of money, so they funded two of the memory bags. It was great to have that link with them. They come in, they borrow them and then you've got that way of passing the information on to families as well. And a big local care company asked me to go into their offices to train their carers who provide a creative intervention for people at home with dementia. They might be doing a four-hour visit to somebody with dementia, so to find that there are resources that can help that they can get from the library was a revelation to them. It's just getting the word out there, isn't it really?
(H. Rodenhurst, conversation with author, 9 November 2021)

This chapter considers some of the ways in which libraries can work in partnership with other organisations to meet the needs of people with dementia. It starts by outlining some established models of partnership working before looking at case studies that illustrate ways of forming partnerships within varied local contexts. The final section focuses on issues around developing partnerships with care homes. This sector is obviously important when developing services for people with dementia and carers, but it can be one of the more challenging for libraries to make inroads into. Drawing on experiences from successful projects, this chapter outlines some suggestions that may be helpful in this respect.

General partnership schemes

Established partnership schemes that bring together local or regional organisations interested in supporting people with dementia and their carers exist in numerous countries. Many libraries are members of these types of partnership schemes to help to work towards a dementia-friendly community in their locality.

Local Dementia Action Alliances

In the UK many library services are part of Local Dementia Action Alliances (LDAAs). There are similar organisations in other countries, such as local dementia alliances in Australia. An LDAA is a group of people representing different sectors within an area who have come together to create a dementia-friendly community alongside local people affected by dementia. An LDAA can be established at any level: a village, city, county or region. There are over 300 LDAAs in the UK. To sign up as a member, a group or organisation has to complete a simple action plan. The action areas chosen by each LDAA are different, reflecting the specific needs of the local community (DAA, 2022).

Members of an LDAA might typically include local businesses; community groups; faith groups; schools and colleges; libraries; museums; shopping centres; charities; and health and social care providers. Any organisation can get involved provided they are able to demonstrate their commitment to supporting people with dementia. Being a member of an LDAA gives a library access to advice and support from other organisations; an opportunity to share ideas; and a space to publicise, and gain support for, library activities for people with dementia and their carers.

Safe Places

Safe Places (www.safeplaces.org.uk) is another UK national scheme that some libraries are part of. This scheme is not just for people with dementia; it encourages businesses and services to provide initial support to anyone who feels lost and vulnerable when out and about in their community. An individual who is feeling vulnerable, scared, confused or lost can ask for help at a Safe Place. This might include people who have learning disabilities or difficulties for instance, as well as people with dementia. A Safe Place is indicated by a sticker displayed prominently in the window of each business or service that has agreed to take on this role. Users of the scheme carry a Safe Place card that they can show at the Safe Place if they need help.

Library-specific partnership schemes

Whilst libraries can play an important role in more general partnership schemes such as LDAAs and Safe Places, there is often a need to develop more specific library-related partnerships and collaborations that involve the library working with one or more partners with an explicit focus on library services, such as information provision.

Partnering on information provision: Memory Connection Center, Wisconsin, US

Whilst library staff are not expected to be dementia experts, libraries can play an important role in the provision of information about dementia through working in partnership with other services. The North Shore Library Memory Connection Center in Wisconsin in the US provides quick access to services, information and support for those caring for individuals with dementia. Some people may be hesitant to go to the district's Aging and Disability Resource Center, so Memory Connection Centers are designed to make gaining access to critical and timely information easy and less intimidating in a place that is accessible and neutral. The aim of this approach is to eliminate the stigma that might be associated with the process of investigating and gaining information about dementia. Library staff receive in-depth training from key community partners regarding warning signs of dementia; the types and stages of dementia; communication strategies;

cultural sensitivity; transportation; and caregiver concerns. They also receive training on the resources available to assist families and how to access them. The goal is for the library to serve as an initial point of access for information and resources. Multiple partners are involved in the Memory Connection Center and library staff work closely with community partners to ensure that the most accurate and highest quality information is provided.

Melody Schuetz, Head of Adult Services at North Shore Library, describes the importance of partnerships in the development of this service:

> The biggest piece of advice I have is to make connections with your community's local department on aging. We collaborated with the Milwaukee County Division on Aging to create the Memory Connection Center about four years ago and continue to work with them now. We have been working with Dementia Care Specialists from the Division on Aging for a few years now. They have offered regular presentations to the public at the library about brain health, dementia care and recognising the signs of dementia, as well as trained our library staff on how to work with people with dementia. Library staff are trained on how to direct patrons to the Memory Connection Center, explain how it works and locate resources. We also train our library staff on recognising patrons with dementia and best practices for serving people with dementia. We've reached out to our county's Division on Aging for assistance with these trainings.
>
> The Dementia Care Specialists have also offered free brain health screenings at the library, which have been popular among our patrons. We've really benefited by this relationship with the Dementia Care Specialists. Last year, for example, we had a library staff member who had been working with a homebound patron to schedule book deliveries. During one of their interactions, the patron insisted that she had scheduled pickup for a certain time and was furious that the staff member had the wrong time. The staff member was certain that she and the patron had agreed on a different time and that the patron was remembering incorrectly. Due to my training with the Division on Aging, I suspected that this patron had dementia and this behaviour was a result of the disease. I arranged a training session for the library staff member with a Dementia Care Specialist and she received some wonderful tips on how to have a successful interaction with that patron. We are still offering homebound delivery service to that patron today and our interactions with her have been much more successful.
>
> (M. Schuetz, e-mail to author, 16 November 2021)

Co-location with other services

Whilst many partnerships, such as that at North Shore Library, are built around the provision of a service or activity, another important form of partnership is the co-location of services. Chapter 3 described several dementia-friendly libraries that are co-located with other services, including leisure and health facilities, a children's centre and a care home. These case studies highlight some of the benefits, but also the challenges, of co-locating with other services. In particular, the importance of ensuring that a building in not simply dementia-friendly in an overall sense, but also that all co-located services are dementia friendly in their own right. Co-located services can offer the convenience of access to several services in one location and have the potential to support broader initiatives, such as intergenerational provision. Co-location can also mean that staff develop a better understanding of the roles of other services in supporting people with dementia and reflect on how they might work together more effectively. However, it is important to consider how co-locating a facility impacts on a customer's experience of the library, particularly those customers who have dementia. For example, it can be more difficult to control acoustics in a co-located facility.

Partnering with care homes

Care homes (whether they provide nursing and/or residential care) are likely to be one of the key partners libraries want to engage with when developing services for people with dementia and their carers. However, it can be challenging to develop partnerships with this sector; there are issues that can make partnering with care homes particularly complex. The first factor is the nature of the sector: whilst there are companies, or local authorities, that manage several homes within an area, the sheer number of care home providers means there is no easy way for a library to reach all local care homes, so partnerships have to be developed on a piecemeal basis, which is obviously time-consuming. Staffing can be another factor: many care homes have high staff-turnover and often lack staffing capacity or specialist staff (for example, not all will have full-time activity co-ordinators). A further factor to consider when working with care homes is that not all staff will have experience or understanding of the role of arts-based or cultural activities, such as reading, in supporting residents. Staff are usually able to appreciate the value of social engagement activities, but arts-related concepts may feel less familiar.

The following examples outline some of the challenges that libraries can face when engaging with care homes, and suggest potential solutions.

Guernsey Libraries' Tovertafel: focus on outreach

It is possible for a library to partner with a care home that wishes to bring some of their residents to the library or to encourage carers to visit and borrow resources. However, outreach activities, delivered within the care home, may be a more realistic option – and be more enthusiastically received by care homes. Jackie Burgess, Community and Outreach Librarian on the island of Guernsey, explains some of the reasons for this in relation to the library's Tovertafel (magic table), described in Chapter 6. She found that, whilst the technology itself is clearly beneficial, dealing with logistical issues around getting people with dementia to a fixed location to use the magic table was challenging.

She concludes that, for Guernsey Libraries, a portable magic table that can be used as part of library outreach activities would be a more practical option for care homes, allowing the library to support care home residents more effectively and meaning more people could benefit from using the technology.

> We used to have regular groups visiting the library to use the Tovertafel, but after a while, they've petered out. The feedback is that care homes are so short of staff and so short of time that they can't physically do it; they can't physically bring all their residents to use the Tovertafel. Obviously Covid hasn't helped; the care homes have been more careful about taking their residents out. Getting residents out and driven to the community library seems to be the difficulty that we've got. I wish the Tovertafel was mobile as I would like to take it to the people in the different nursing homes and care homes.
>
> (J. Burgess, conversation with author, 24 November 2021)

Halton Libraries' reminiscence boxes: emphasising the value of the library offer

At Halton library service in the UK, staff have run reminiscence sessions in care homes using themed reminiscence boxes for several years. Box contents include photographs from Halton's local history collection, along with physical objects and books such as the *Pictures to Share* range (see Chapter 4) and local history books. Prior to starting the reminiscence box service, the outreach team had been attempting to fill the gap left by the closure of the mobile library service by taking books and other lending items to care homes in much the same way as the mobile library had done. However, as they visited care homes and sheltered accommodation, they started discussing the needs of the residents in more detail with residents themselves, care staff, activity co-ordinators and managers. They realised that, although the mobile service had been popular, the library service was not reaching many care home residents. What those individuals needed more than book lending was enriching face-to-face activities. This prompted the outreach team to develop a more engaged reminiscence box model delivering group sessions on a regular basis in a number of homes. The staff would bring reminiscence boxes on a variety of themes, such as childhood, school days, sport and women. The box contents were selected by library staff, using their professional and local knowledge to select items with local significance. Whilst library staff bring their expertise in resource selection and the resources themselves, care home staff taking part would know the residents' individual needs and ways of interacting. They also knew about residents' backgrounds and personal histories, so were able to use this knowledge to encourage them to participate in the sessions.

Trudy Jones, Library Development Officer at Halton Libraries, describes the value of working closely with care home staff and some of the challenges they have faced both before and since COVID-19:

> Obviously, the care home staff know their residents really well, so it's a real benefit to have them in the sessions. For example, there was a gentleman in one home who had been a farmer. He used to just sit there in the sessions. So we bought some picture books with farm machinery and that kind of thing and I sat and asked him if any of these machines looked familiar. And he started this big conversation about the

farming year and which crops they grew. His face lit up because somebody was actually talking about something he knew about. So having staff supporting you in that way can be really helpful and make the sessions really rewarding.

Initially, we had problems because we would turn up at the home and the staff would have completely forgotten that we were coming, so they would scramble a few people together. We felt that if we were going to do this, we needed reliable support from them. So, after a couple of occasions with that happening, we thought, 'Hang on, we need to get this more structured; we need them to value our service'. So we would remind them we were coming and then if they forgot a couple of times, we said, 'Sorry, we're not going be able to give you the service anymore'. When we did that, they replied quickly and said, 'Oh, we're really sorry, but we'll definitely have someone ready next time'.

One of the other problems we had was that it varied as to how involved the activity co-ordinator was. We had a couple who were absolutely brilliant. They asked people to get photos to bring to the session and things like that, and really got involved in the session and practically ran it themselves. But we had other situations where people would see it as, 'Oh, good, the library's coming in; we can go and check out some paperwork'. Even though we've all had quite a lot of training in dementia, we're not experts, so I felt that it was putting us in a vulnerable position. And it's about the comfort of people taking part as well: if they want to use the toilet during a session and that kind of thing. So again, we had to put our foot down and say, 'There must be a member of staff with us, or we won't be able to do it'. After that, people were available for us. But I think, again, it's about putting over the value of what we're offering, because they're free sessions, so making the care homes realise that they're getting quite a lot really.

Obviously, we couldn't go into care homes once Covid started. For about the first nine months, we offered them a few online things such as quizzes and we signed up to a database of photographs they could use. But it very much depended on whether the activity co-ordinator had to cover for other staff with personal care and so on. But then we started to deliver a memory box to each care home every month. We pooled our resources, so in each memory box we've got a clearly set out plan for a member of staff to use to run a session themselves. We used to do a poem at the beginning and end of a session, so we've put those in too. They've said it's great because it gives them something different to do because activities were pushed to one side in a lot of places. We also took the opportunity to go to all the care homes that we hadn't engaged with before and a couple of them have taken us up on the monthly reminiscence box service.

(T. Jones, conversation with author, 18 January 2022)

Trudy offered the following advice for other library services considering offering a similar service to care homes:

- Be fairly structured in how you plan the sessions – you'll likely be asked to fill a slot in between other activities or to fit into a regular schedule so you'll need to stick to that.
- Getting to the right person is important. If you can get through to the manager, then that's a good starting point, and find out if they've got an activity co-ordinator. We have a good health improvement team in Halton who have created a group for activity co-ordinators, so that's useful. There's also a local care home managers' meeting that happens regularly, so I go along to that to speak to them.

- Going to the home and taking a memory box is better than trying to explain to someone over the phone.
- Laying down the ground rules is important, such as saying you will only be able to do it with a member of staff present.
- You've got to persevere because when you mention the word library, you've then got to explain why you might be relevant to them and what you can offer. Usually people are pleasantly surprised!
- Everyone on the team delivering the sessions had quite a bit of dementia training, such as Dementia Friends, and we tend to go to any development opportunities to do with dementia. That has helped a lot because at first it's quite daunting, particularly if people are non-verbal.

Words in Mind, Kirklees: offering staff training

Many of the challenges faced by Halton Libraries' reminiscence box service were also experienced by Words in Mind (see Chapter 4), a successful bibliotherapy project run by people with considerable expertise in, and experience of, partnership working. Nevertheless, engaging staff in care homes was particularly challenging. Where there was a dedicated activity co-ordinator who understood and supported the project, it was much easier, but not all care homes had someone in this role. The care homes where the type of intervention offered by Words in Mind might perhaps make the greatest impact were often precisely those lacking members of staff who could offer the support required to ensure the success of sessions.

Although there was a service level agreement in place between Words in Mind and each partner organisation, staff in a number of care homes did not appear clear about levels of support or involvement required; for example, the need for staff from the home to attend sessions to support residents and use their knowledge of the group members (for example, their hobbies and family life) to prompt greater involvement. Care home staff appeared to be supportive of the project and enthusiastic about the overall benefits of participating for their residents, but were not always aware of the practicalities of a session.

To try to improve understanding of bibliotherapy within the care homes involved, Words in Mind offered training to their staff. This was similar to the training offered to the volunteers and sessional workers who led the Words in Mind sessions. Not all staff attended, but for those who did, the training led to more active involvement in sessions from care home staff. The Words in Mind sessions are probably a little different from activities many care home staff are used to, so it required additional support and training to develop greater understanding of what the project was aiming to achieve and to help staff to understand how they might best support a session and encourage residents to attend.

Sefton Library Service's Lost Voices project: the importance of ongoing communication

A common problem faced by libraries working with care homes can be trying to identify those residents who could benefit most from the service or resource being offered. It is important to ensure care home staff are clear about the types of residents who are likely to benefit from taking part in an activity. Of course, this varies from activity to activity and some have a much wider target audience than others.

Lesley Davies, Senior Development Manager at Sefton Library Services, describes some challenges faced by the Lost Voices project (see Chapter 5). Whilst reminiscence activities are likely to be more familiar to care home staff than arts-based or bibliotherapy initiatives, it is still important to communicate regularly with care homes and emphasise the importance of taking care when identifying people for a particular activity.

> Sometimes our volunteers have been sent into residents' rooms and they've started trying to have a conversation, but it just hasn't been possible to get anything meaningful. The volunteers will come back to me and say it's upsetting for them because they're trying to press people to remember and they're struggling because their dementia is more advanced. So I've had to go in to the care homes (and sometimes it's a difficult conversation to have) to say, 'We need to have people who can remember things and we can't put our volunteers in a position where they're feeling that they're upsetting people by trying to record'. So we've had a couple of difficult conversations. I would always go in before we started working and try and explain that. But sometimes, if the activity co-ordinator has changed in the time between when I've been in and we started recording, that message might have been lost. But we do quite firmly say, 'Participants have to be able to hold a conversation and still have those memories to make it meaningful for the person, their family and us'. We're doing it for the benefit of the people who are having the recordings and their family.
>
> (L. Davies, conversation with author, 1 April 2022)

Describing library activities in 'care sector language'

As discussed above, some care staff may initially find it difficult to relate to, or see the potential benefits of, services offered by the library for people with dementia or carers. Whilst their training and experiences are likely to mean they recognise the benefits of more social- or reminiscence-focused activities, the concepts underpinning cultural or arts-focused activities may be less familiar.

To help care staff more easily understand the need for, and appreciate the potential benefits of, some library activities for people with dementia, it may therefore be worth reflecting on the language used to describe the activities. Several of the case studies presented in this book are described in terms of Tom Kitwood's model of person-centred care. The same approach could be taken with other library activities or services. The benefit of describing activities in this way is that the language is more likely to be familiar to social care professionals than 'library language'. They may therefore be able to appreciate the benefits offered more clearly – and, if necessary, present it to their own managers or colleagues in a context that demonstrates how partnering with a library service can support high quality dementia care.

An example is the Reading is Caring project (described in Chapter 4). In this project, the creation of 'life story book boxes' was deliberately linked to ideas from life story work that would be familiar to most care staff. Life story work 'involves working with a person with dementia, family members and friends to record key moments of their past and present lives' (SCIE, 2020d) and often involves the creation of a 'memory box' of special items from their life. Reading is Caring extended this familiar idea to create a book box of reading materials, as well as objects that had meaning for the person.

Many successful collaborative projects – across a range of sectors – empathise the importance of having someone who can 'interpret' between collaborators from different sectors to overcome barriers presented by language used by professionals from different backgrounds (for example, Martynova et al., 2020). While this is not always possible in practice, libraries can help to secure a higher level of engagement and buy-in from care staff by presenting ideas using terms that are likely to be more familiar within the care sector, even if they are not 'fluent' in that language.

Conclusions

Partnership working is essential in the provision of library services for people with dementia and their carers. Of course, library staff are not expected to be experts in dementia, so it is vital to involve partners who can bring that expertise when designing and delivering new services, activities or buildings. Depending on the activities or services offered, libraries may also benefit from partnerships with individuals or organisations with expertise in other areas, such as design, the arts or technology. Whilst some partnerships are relatively easy to facilitate, others can be more challenging, especially if the organisation involved does not have a history of working with library services.

This chapter has focused most attention on care homes as this can be one of the more challenging sectors for libraries to engage with. However, the potential solutions described, such as reinforcing the value of the library's offer, providing staff training opportunities and ensuring there is ongoing communication, would also apply to many other potential partner organisations. As many of the case studies illustrate, language and communication can be an important consideration in building a successful partnership. Chapter 8 considers some of the issues to be aware of in communications about dementia more generally.

8
Communications and Marketing

> The stigmatised images – makes you think that that's all there is – that there's nothing left to look forward to, but they're wrong.
> (Bould, *Dementia-friendly Media and Broadcast Guide*, 2018)

Chapter 2 discussed the importance of reflecting on face-to-face interactions with people with dementia in the library and, if necessary, developing better communication skills to improve their experience of library services. This chapter focuses on communications about the library and its services in written formats, as this is how people with dementia and their carers are initially likely to find out about services available to them through their library. This includes print materials but also, of course, digital communications. In many cases there is room to improve communications. For instance, as research involving Scottish public libraries pointed out, if the public only used library web pages as their source of information, they would not know that many services are dementia friendly as this is rarely mentioned (Tyler, 2020). On the other hand, whilst researching this book, I came across several instances where dementia-friendly services advertised on library websites did not reflect what happened in practice. This included facilities that were advertised as being accessible for people with dementia in promotional materials, but which I was told were not in fact suitable when I enquired about them.

Whilst the guidance below offers some general suggestions to take into consideration when designing marketing and communications materials, it is important to consult with people with dementia, and other groups such as carers, to ensure these meet the needs of local library audiences. Chapter 9 suggests some consultation methods that may be helpful.

This chapter starts with a discussion of some of the key terminology used when discussing dementia. Much of this applies to both written and verbal communication, but it is particularly important in materials promoting library services to ensure that, as far as possible, the ways in which they are described is inclusive of people with dementia and carers. The second section of the chapter focuses on the design of materials intended to be accessible for people with dementia – both in print and online – and also discusses the inclusion of images and considerations such as the translation of resources into community languages.

Language and terminology

Words matter. The words we use, in both speech and writing, can influence the mood, self-esteem and feelings of others. As with any group of people, the language we use to talk about dementia influences how people with the condition are viewed and potentially how they feel about themselves. A casual misuse of words, or the use of words with negative connotations, when talking about dementia in everyday conversations can have a profound impact on someone with dementia, as well as on their family and friends. It can also influence how others think about dementia and increase the likelihood of a person with dementia experiencing stigma or discrimination in their everyday interactions. Using positive language, on the other hand, can make people feel valued and included. Treating people with dignity and respect as individuals through the language used can contribute to changing how society views and treats people with dementia.

Whilst there are some terms that are widely acknowledged to be unhelpful, in other cases, decisions about which words are 'best' is less clear and individual judgement is likely to be needed. For example, the UK Alzheimer's Society (2018) and Dementia Australia (2021b) include 'stressful' as a word that they consider acceptable to use to describe the impact of dementia. However, whilst this may be an appropriate term in some circumstances, I would recommend caution using this in more general communications because, as with more obviously negative terms, it may imply that people are destined to find dementia stressful.

It is worth looking at some key terminology in detail to help to make informed decisions about how to refer to people with dementia and their carers in library publicity and marketing materials.

Person with dementia

While it is important to be realistic about the impact of dementia, as with any situation, using words that are negative, disempowering, pessimistic or frightening is rarely helpful. Throughout this book, the terms 'people with dementia' and 'people living with dementia' are used. When people with dementia are discussed in the media, however, words like 'sufferers' and 'victims' still often appear. Terms such as these are unhelpful as they risk stigmatising people with dementia as a group. Of course, if an individual with dementia chooses to use these sorts of words to describe how they feel about their personal experience of living with the condition, it is important to respect that. However, when talking to, or about, people with dementia collectively, it should not be assumed that this is the case.

Furthermore, language is constantly evolving and there are words to describe dementia that may have been common in the past but are no longer recommended, for example 'demented' or 'senile'. In addition to checking new resources that are created, it is therefore worth reviewing all materials periodically to check that they still comply with current recommendations for language use in relation to dementia.

Another issue to be aware of is that there can sometimes be confusion because a word might be used or understood in different ways. For instance, whilst 'living with dementia' usually refers to a person with dementia themselves, some carers may refer to themselves in this way as they are also affected by the condition. To avoid confusion, the term 'affected by dementia' can be used to refer to a much larger group that includes people with the condition plus their carers, friends, family or anyone else who is close to them or provides support.

For practical reasons general marketing and communication materials about library services usually need to be as all-encompassing as possible, but it is worth remembering that, individually, some people may identify in different ways. For example, some might view themselves as someone with Alzheimer's disease or someone with memory problems, rather than thinking of themselves as a 'person with dementia'. In addition, whilst some people may feel encouraged to take part in an activity that is promoted as explicitly for people with dementia, because they feel confident that measures will be put in place to make sure it is inclusive, others may avoid attending an activity advertised in this way, particularly if they have not had a formal diagnosis or are finding it difficult to come to terms with the fact that they have dementia. Indeed, there may be instances where the person is not aware that they have dementia because their carer wants to keep the diagnosis from them.

Whatever our personal feelings on these situations, it is important to find the most effective ways to promote opportunities to those people who are likely to benefit from them. An example of an inclusive description is that used for Stockton Library's Local History Group, described in Chapter 5. This is advertised as being 'for older people and people living with dementia' and suitable for people who 'are living with dementia or simply need more time and support' (Stockton Information Directory, n.d.). This potentially allows people to see themselves joining the group whether or not they have a diagnosis or think of themselves as a person with dementia.

It is also important to consider cultural differences that may be relevant for some library audiences. For instance, as Kristen Jacklin and colleagues point out in relation to indigenous communities in Canada, although much mainstream practice and current recommendations may suggest steering away from using the term 'loved one' to describe a person with dementia, indigenous partners have expressed that this term is appropriate for use in indigenous communities (Jacklin et al., 2018).

In some cases, for example libraries within healthcare facilities, it may be appropriate to refer to 'dementia patients'; but in libraries outside the healthcare system, avoid referring to people with dementia as 'patients'. Like anyone with a health condition, people with dementia are only patients when they are interacting with healthcare services and professionals.

Carer

The use of the term 'carer' can also bring complexities. Some of those who support a person with dementia might not identify as a carer, especially if the person they are supporting is in the earlier stages of the condition. In the UK the term 'carer' can be used to refer to people who provide unpaid care, such as a partner, family member or friend, as well as those who are employed to care for someone. In other countries, alternative terms, such as 'caregiver', may be more common. In some situations it can be helpful to use different words for paid carers, such as 'care workers' or '(social) care professionals', with unpaid carers being referred to as 'family carers', for example. Furthermore, whilst the terms 'carer' or 'caregiver' are widely accepted and used within social- and health-care settings (for example, in the UK there is a carer's assessment to apply for support and a carer's allowance paid through the benefits system), not everyone likes to be referred to, or even sees themselves, as a carer; they may simply think of themselves as a wife, husband, son, daughter, friend and so forth. For some marketing and communication materials, it may therefore be more appropriate to use a phrase such as 'family and friends' rather than carers. There is no single 'right' approach; the important thing is to find out what terms are likely to engage the audience you want to reach.

A possible alternative term for carer is 'care partner'. This term indicates an agreement between a person with a chronic condition and their family member or friend to be partners in care, as best as they can, and to help each other with health, wellness and caring for each other. However, this term can also be problematic as, to some people, it may imply that it relates only to a person's partner or spouse. In addition, it may not reflect the way in which a carer for someone with more advanced dementia feels about their role.

The term 'loved ones' has become more common in general discourse over the last few decades. Whilst this does have the advantage of encompassing both family members and close friends of someone with dementia, it is not a term everyone feels comfortable with, especially if the past relationship between the person with dementia and their family or friends may have been problematic.

There are links to further resources and guidance about language and dementia in the annotated bibliography. However, the language used in communications and marketing materials is not the only factor to consider. It is also important to ensure the needs of people with dementia are taken into account in the way in which library publicity materials are designed.

Design of communications materials

Basic principles of plain language and good design are especially important in the design of publicity or communications materials aimed at people with dementia. It is also crucial that people with dementia are consulted about the accessibility of published materials. As a basic framework to consider the needs of people with dementia, the '7Cs of communication' may be helpful. These state that the materials should consider each of the following points:

1 **Correct:** as well as being factually correct, the terms you use need to be suited to your audience – use words people are likely to use themselves.
2 **Complete:** include all relevant information – contact names, dates, times, locations, etc., including information that people with dementia may need to be aware of (for example, support available).
3 **Concrete:** make sure your audience has a clear picture of what you're telling them; information and actions required should be clear so the reader knows what they need to do.
4 **Concise:** are there any adjectives or 'filler words' that you can delete to make the communication clearer?
5 **Coherent:** ensure all points are connected and relevant to the main topic and that the tone and flow of the text are consistent.
6 **Courteous:** be empathetic to people's needs and treat people with dementia with respect.

7 **Clear:** try to minimise the number of ideas in each sentence; people should not have to read between the lines and make assumptions to understand what you are trying to say.

When designing materials, it is important to make sure that the flow of information is clear, so people know what order they are expected to read a document in. A consistent layout throughout a document is helpful, as is highlighting the most important information, for example by using bold font. Finish sentences on the same page where they begin so that readers do not omit to turn the page, particularly in the case of instructions and disclaimers.

In addition to layout, the amount of information provided in materials intended to be read by people with dementia is another consideration. Try to ensure that reading does not require long periods of concentration. This means considering the amount of text both in the document overall and on each page or section. Breaking up detailed information into shorter sections that can be read individually can be helpful. Use bullet points, bold text, titles and headings to present information in manageable sections.

The broad principles discussed above apply to online, as well as print, materials. Websites also need to be easy to navigate and not overload the reader with information.

The annotated bibliography includes links to more specific design guidance that may be helpful to share with designers when creating materials intended to be inclusive for people with dementia. However, it is important to be realistic; no single format is guaranteed to meet everyone's needs.

Images

The importance of images in publicity and communications materials should not be overlooked. Images can be useful to reinforce written information. For example, including photographs in a leaflet describing library services can be helpful so that people know what to expect when they arrive.

However, images often used in resources for people with dementia can perpetuate negative stereotypes of the condition, for instance a fading face or wrinkled hands. Resources such as the Centre for Ageing Better's age-positive image library (https://ageingbetter.resourcespace.com/pages/home.php) can be useful to help identify more positive images, but also try to involve people with dementia themselves in the selection, or creation, of images.

Generally, more abstract images may be difficult for a person with dementia to interpret, so simple clear illustrations or photographs tend to work best. Also, avoid overlaying text on images as this can make writing more difficult to read.

Translations

In some cases libraries may wish to translate information about services for people with dementia into community languages. Whilst this is undoubtedly helpful in potentially expanding access to services, care and expert advice is needed. Words and phrases that are appropriate in one language may be offensive, ambiguous or meaningless in another. Specifically, in some languages there is no equivalent word for dementia and in some cases the closest words can imply 'madness'. Again, the involvement of members of the target audience in the design of materials can be invaluable in highlighting where a literal translation is not the most appropriate and a more nuanced approach is needed.

Working with the media and other partners

Links with media outlets, such as a local newspaper or radio station, can be invaluable in helping to publicise library services and especially in attracting new customers. However, a word of warning from experience: if you are working with the media or another communications partner, make sure you have sight of the final copy if possible. It is not always feasible of course, but it can be useful as many media and communications outlets do not currently base their communications about dementia on guidelines such as those described in this chapter. You may find they use terms that you might want to challenge and suggest alternatives for. The UK Alzheimer's Society produces a *Dementia-friendly Media and Broadcast Guide* (Bould, 2018), which may be useful when working with media partners.

It is also important to build up a relationship with other local partners so that you can suggest changes to their communication materials if necessary. For example, when visiting libraries that are promoted as being dementia friendly, I have seen leaflets or flyers advertising local services that use terms such as 'dementia sufferers'. Although these materials are not produced by the library itself, the distinction may not be obvious to customers and could impact on their perception of the library as a dementia-friendly location.

Conclusions

This chapter has highlighted the complexities of designing marketing and communications materials that are inclusive of people with dementia and their carers. Whilst guidelines such as those included in the annotated bibliography are useful, it is vital to include people with dementia and their carers directly in communications design. Chapter 9 focuses on evaluation and service development and suggests a range of methods that can be used to engage people with dementia and their carers in order to gather their feedback on library communications materials – as well as other aspects of library provision for people with dementia.

9
Evaluation and Service Development

> Having a person living with dementia audit the library with a member of staff means it's not just the librarian saying, 'Yes, our signage looks okay'.
> (Heather Cowie, National Project Manager, Dementia-Friendly Canada, in conversation with author)

Most library staff understand the importance of evaluating their services in order to develop and improve the levels of service and types of provision they offer to customers. However, many of the methods commonly used to gather user feedback on library services are not well-suited to the needs of people with dementia. This chapter explores ways in which libraries can ensure that the views of people with dementia and their carers can be taken into account in their evaluation, research and service development activities.

The chapter starts by outlining key concepts to consider, based on Tom Kitwood's model of person-centred care, which was described in detail in Chapter 1. It also discusses why it is important to involve both carers and people with dementia directly in evaluation activities. This is followed by descriptions of research and evaluation methods, including interviews, focus groups and visual methods, outlining how, with some adaptations or extra considerations, they can be effectively used to gather feedback from people with dementia, as well as their carers. The chapter finishes by reflecting on some of the ethical issues that need to be taken into account when undertaking research generally and with people with dementia in particular.

The aim of this chapter is to focus on aspects of evaluation and service development that are most important to consider when working with people with dementia. There are links to more general guidance on research and evaluation methods in the annotated bibliography.

Key concepts

As outlined in Chapter 2, a dementia-friendly business or service 'is responsive to the needs of people affected by dementia and makes efforts to understand the impact of dementia in their community by ensuring that people living with dementia and their care partners are included and consulted in conversations about becoming dementia friendly' (Alzheimer Society of Saskatchewan, 2019, 4). If a library wishes to be dementia friendly, it is important that it involves both people with dementia and their carers in decisions about new services or about changes to existing library provision. This includes services explicitly aimed at people with dementia, as well as more general developments that are likely to affect all library customers.

It is important to stress that people with dementia and their carers are important audiences to consider and that their views may differ. Whilst feedback from carers is crucial to understand better the impact of the library service on their experiences, it is important to bear in mind that feedback about the impact of services on quality of life from carers may (quite reasonably) reflect the carer's own needs and quality of life, rather than what matters most to the person with dementia. Whilst carers can, of course, be effective advocates for people with dementia, research has shown that often carers (or other proxies) may perceive quality of life and experience very differently to people with dementia and often more negatively (O'Shea et al., 2020). This underlines the importance of using dementia-friendly methods and environments to involve people with dementia directly wherever possible and not only rely on talking with others about them.

A further factor to be mindful of is that the term 'carer' can include both paid carers and family members or friends who support a person with dementia. When evaluating library provision, it is therefore important to consider which type(s) of carer you should involve as they may have quite different needs and expectations. This decision depends on the nature of the services in question and who is the target audience.

When involving people with dementia as participants in evaluation or research activities, the model developed by Tom Kitwood (1997) provides a useful basis through which to consider the suitability of different methods and approaches. Table 9.1 opposite sets out some brief pointers, which are expanded on in the sections that follow.

Recruiting participants

The first question to consider if you want to involve people with dementia and their carers in evaluation or research activities is: how are you going to recruit participants? Recruiting from existing library customers is often the

Table 9.1 *Key evaluation concepts mapped onto Kitwood's model*

Comfort	• Welcome participants and make sure they have everything they need. • Make sure the setting is somewhere that people will feel comfortable – ideally somewhere they are used to being. • Make sure the activity is something that everyone can feel they can be involved in or achieve.
Occupation	• Emphasise that you appreciate the time and insights people are giving and explain how you intend to use the information gathered. Follow up on this to explain what has happened as a result of their input in an accessible way (regardless of whether you think the person will remember their involvement). • Be flexible in your approach to suit the needs of different individuals involved.
Attachment	• Whilst you will sometimes need to conduct one-off evaluation activities, try to develop ongoing relationships where possible to build connections with the library. • Provide support for people with dementia, but make sure that any carers present don't 'take over' the session. Getting the balance right can sometimes be tricky
Identity	• Emphasise the role of people with dementia as experts in this context who you want to learn from. • It may be possible to make connections between activities people have done in the past and an evaluation. For instance, someone who was a union representative or had a health and safety role at work may feel a sense of familiarity completing checklists to evaluate library premises.
Inclusion	• Provide different options to make sure everyone feels included – this may mean adopting a greater variety of methods than you might have anticipated. • Including non-verbal methods can be particularly useful.

most straightforward option. This might be done informally, especially in a smaller library, or by contacting customers via e-mail, social media or posters in the library. If there is a regular activity, such as a memory café, held in the library, it may be possible to recruit participants from this group and even include the evaluation activity as part of one of their regular sessions so that people do not have to make a special journey.

Chapter 8 explored some of the issues around how language is used in communication materials targeted towards people with dementia or their carers. A particular concern for evaluation activities, however, is whether you want to recruit *only* people with dementia and/or carers (for example, to gather feedback on a proposed service specifically for that group) or whether you want to make sure people with dementia are included as part of a broader evaluation activity (such as a library refurbishment). In some ways the latter can be more challenging as you need to make sure that people with dementia know their input will be welcomed and feel confident they will be able to take part in whatever activity is proposed and contribute effectively. In practice, this might mean explicitly targeting people with dementia and explaining the evaluation and what they will be asked to do in greater detail than might be considered necessary for library customers more generally.

Of course, recruiting from existing library customers limits the pool of possible participants. One way to widen the range of participants is to work with an external organisation, such as a local dementia support group or advocacy organisation, in order to recruit from a broader group that they have access to. In the UK the Alzheimer's Society has a dementia directory that can help to identify useful local services (www.alzheimers.org.uk/find-support-near-you).

Evaluation and research methods

There are a variety of ways to gather data on library services. Decisions about which method(s) to use depend, to a large extent, on two factors: (1) the target audience you wish to participate in the evaluation; and (2) the questions you wish to answer through the evaluation.

Surveys

Surveys are probably the most common evaluation method in libraries. Questionnaires are undoubtedly useful if you want to conduct research with a large sample and generalise the findings to a wider population. They are helpful if you want to confirm, or refute, a hypothesis, but can be less suited to more complex questions (for example, if you want to ask 'Does this approach work?', but not '*How* does this approach work?').

For carers, questionnaires can be an effective way to gather data as they can be completed any time, fitted around other commitments and usually done anywhere, meaning there is no need to organise respite care. However, it is important to be aware that, while an online survey may be preferred by some carers, it would naturally be tricky for those without internet access or digital skills. Having both an online and print option may therefore be helpful as this brings flexibility.

It is also possible to design a questionnaire suitable for people with dementia, especially those in the early stages of the condition, but this takes care and it is unlikely to be the best method to involve many people with dementia. If you want to design a written questionnaire suitable for people with dementia, follow the general advice provided in Chapter 8 about written communication materials. Some additional suggestions specifically for questionnaire design are as follows:

1 Try to keep the format of questions as standardised as possible. If you ask questions with several different scales (for example, important–unimportant *and* agree–disagree) this can get confusing.
2 Limit the number of different types of questions you ask. For example, a scale question, followed by a ranking question, followed by a 'choose the top 3' question can become confusing.
3 As far as possible, limit the number of options you offer in multiple choice or scale questions to three or four options.
4 If you include open questions, make sure that you provide sufficient space for someone to write their answer. In online surveys, answer boxes are often limited to three lines and the text scrolls up as you write more. A larger response box is better so the respondent can see the whole of their answer as they write.
5 As with any survey, do not use questions that require respondents to reply with a double negative, for example, 'I didn't enjoy my visit to the library' (that confuses too many people for the findings to be valid for almost any target audience!).
6 It is a good idea to avoid overly long questionnaires for any audience, but especially for people with dementia who may well take longer to answer.
7 Pilot the questionnaire with members of the group you are expecting to answer it (that is, people with dementia or their carers). For people with dementia, you may find it more effective to carry out piloting face-to-face (rather than asking for written feedback at the end) so that they can explain what they are thinking as they go through the questionnaire. Check how long they take to complete the questionnaire; for the majority of questionnaires it should ideally be less than five minutes and certainly no more than ten.

If you want to carry out a survey with people with dementia, a written questionnaire is not your only option. An alternative is a short face-to-face survey. In this scenario, someone reads questions aloud and writes the answers given by the respondent. This means that the person with dementia can ask for clarification if necessary and is not left 'stranded' because they are unsure how to answer a question. In this case, it is best to keep to a limited number of questions (eight to ten maximum), and to make sure that the person with dementia has a print copy to read and keep track of what is being asked.

Interviews

There are several options when conducting interviews with a person with dementia and it is important to try to adopt the approach that feels most comfortable to the person involved, as far as possible. Some people with dementia, especially in the early stages, may be happy to be interviewed alone; others may prefer to be with a carer who can support them. The latter option can work well but may sometimes be problematic if the carer places more emphasis on their own views rather than advocating on behalf of the person with dementia. A third alternative is for a small number of people with dementia to be interviewed together to provide peer support for each other. This can also remove the pressure if an individual is struggling to think of an answer. Although researchers use the term 'interview', when explaining what is involved to members of the public, I typically use more everyday terms such as 'chat'.

What is an interview?

There are several types of research interview. Semi-structured interviews are probably the most common approach. This type of interview is based around a number of predetermined open-ended questions. However, the wording and order of these questions can be altered by the interviewer to make the conversation flow more naturally or to use terms the interviewee is most familiar with. In addition, the interviewer may ask follow-up questions, prompted by the interviewees' responses to the initial questions.

Alternatively, in narrative, or unstructured, interviews, the interviewer does not have a guide to structure their questioning. Instead, there is a predetermined focus for the interview, and the interviewer asks whatever questions they feel will help them to achieve the overall aims of their research. This type of interviewing generally requires greater skill on the part of the interviewer, as well as an in-depth understanding of the topic they are researching. Narrative interviews tend to feel more like a natural conversation and it is important that the interviewer builds up a rapport with the interviewee – often over the course of a series of meetings. This process of developing a relationship and degree of understanding between interviewer and interviewee, and less concern about diverging from the pre-determined questions, may be a useful one to consider when involving people with dementia in research.

Another approach is to think about the interview as a reciprocal, collaborative process. Conversational interviews attempt to address the hierarchical power relationship that can occur in other forms of interviewing where the interviewer has considerably more control of the process than the interviewee. Building a rapport with the interviewee is important in establishing trust, respect and empathy. Rather than attempting to remain detached and objective, the interviewer may become more personally involved in the interview, for example, sharing their own experiences in response to issues discussed. This type of interview may be useful to consider for gathering data from carers who may want to share their experiences – and potentially offload frustrations they might feel – in a more informal way.

Arranging the interview

People with dementia may feel more confident using certain forms of communication than others, so offer interviewees a range of communication options (for example, phone, e-mail, text, post) so that they can make arrangements in a way that suits them best. Also, be aware that in some cases you may need to make arrangements to meet the person via, or in conjunction with, their carer. In any event, it is helpful to send a reminder a day or two before and on the day of the interview itself. Understand that people may need to drop out at short notice for a number of reasons and it is better for both the interviewee and the research itself if the interview is rearranged for a time when they feel better able to participate.

Where at all possible, the interview should take place somewhere familiar to the participant. When this is not possible, it should at least be a type of location where they are likely to feel comfortable; for example, a formal boardroom may feel intimidating to many people. Whether or not the interviewee has visited the location before, provide them with detailed instructions, ideally including images of the building; contact details in case of delays or problems; and instructions for what to do once they arrive, for example where the reception is and who to ask for. The location used for the interview needs to be private and reasonably quiet so that the interview can be conducted without distractions. However, there is no need to stick to conventional locations: ask the interviewee where they would prefer to be interviewed (or give them options). For example, walking whilst being interviewed can help the process to seem more natural and comfortable for some people.

Conducting interviews by phone or online is another option that avoids the need for travel or respite care. Indeed, this can often be a convenient option for carers. Obviously online interviews rely on the interviewee having internet access and feeling comfortable with video conferencing, but one positive outcome of the COVID-19 pandemic is that more people are now used to this type of technology. Phone or online interviews may also work for someone with dementia, especially those in the early stages of the condition. However, face-to-face interactions where they have more opportunities to pick up on body language and other communication cues are likely to make the process easier.

When planning your interview, you should decide on a time that is most convenient for the participant and takes account of the daily patterns of their life. Try to find out when the interviewee feels they are likely to be able to concentrate best and are least likely to be worrying about other things they have to do.

Conducting the interview

Many of the tips for communicating with people with dementia outlined in Chapter 2 will apply when conducting an interview. In particular, the following points may be helpful – most of these are simply good interview practice in any situation but are particularly important when interviewing someone with dementia:

1. Sit where the person can see and hear you as clearly as possible.
2. Listen carefully to what the person is saying. Offer encouragement both verbally and non-verbally, for example by making eye contact and nodding.
3. Allow the person plenty of time to respond – it may take them a little longer to process the information and work out their response. They may also respond in a more indirect way, giving themselves time to think through their answer, so make sure you give them time and encouragement to go through that process.
4. If the person does not understand a question, even after you repeat it, try asking it in a slightly different way instead. If they still do not understand, move onto the next question – you can return to the initial question later if appropriate.
5. If you have not fully understood what the person has said, ask them to repeat it. If you are still unclear, rephrase their answer to check your understanding of what they meant.
6. Try to stick to one idea at a time and avoid asking multiple questions at once.
7. If a person with dementia is accompanied by a carer in the interview, make sure you speak directly to the person with dementia rather than only focusing on the person they are with.

The use of images and objects as stimulus material – for example photographs, diagrams, maps, timelines, film, collage and drawings – can be particularly useful in interviews with people with dementia. This is discussed further under 'visual methods' below.

Emotional touchpoints

An example of the use of stimulus material in an interview is 'emotional touchpoints'. A touchpoint is any point of contact when a user interacts in some way with a service. The aim of this activity is to identify the moments where the person recalls being touched emotionally (feelings) or cognitively (deep and lasting memories). Two sets of cards are used that can include words, images or both (for an example, see www.hisengage.scot/media/1745/emotional-touchpoint-cards.pdf).

- *Touchpoint cards* identify particular aspects of service delivery or practice that you want to learn more about, for example 'taking out a library book'. For each one, you should prepare a card. Have blank cards so that you can add other touchpoints when you are using the cards with a customer.
- *Emotional experience* cards have an emotion on them such as 'happy', 'angry', 'sad' or 'pleased'. Have blank cards in this set too, so that you can add other emotions as necessary.

Show the person whose story you are gathering with the touchpoint cards and encourage them to select one they would like to talk about. You can also offer them the option to talk about a different touchpoint of their own choosing, using one of your blank cards to note this new touchpoint. For each touchpoint you look at together, ask the person to choose emotion cards that match their experience – or to add new words (using the blank cards). Depending on the person you are working with, you may want to limit the number of cards you offer them to choose between to make the process more manageable. Once they have chosen a card, ask them why they selected it. Also ask them to choose a card that shows how they would ideally like to feel. Then ask them what they think would help them to feel this way.

Walking interviews

Walking interviews can be especially useful if you are interested in issues connected with place, an obvious example being the design or layout of a library building. This form of interviewing involves the interviewer accompanying an interviewee around a particular location, whilst observing how they interact with the environment and asking questions. There are different ways to carry out a walking interview: the interviewee may guide the interviewer around a location (this can be a familiar location or an unfamiliar one); alternatively, the interviewer may accompany the interviewee on a trip they regularly make. Sometimes, walking interviews can include travel by other forms of transport (for example, a journey on public transport). In some walking interviews, video or still images are used to record features of the route taken.

An alternative, more structured, approach is to ask one or more participants to fill in (or respond verbally to) a checklist as they walk around a space such as a library. A number of organisations have produced checklists to assess the dementia friendliness of public spaces that could be used for this activity; you can find details in the annotated bibliography.

Focus groups

Another possible method to involve people with dementia or their carers in research and evaluation is a focus group or group discussion. In a focus group, a group of people are asked a series of questions based around a loose topic guide. The topic guide allows for variation, for example in the order in which questions are asked and the inclusion of additional prompts by the facilitator. This may sound very similar to an interview; however, focus groups are most concerned with the interaction between group participants, rather than between the interviewer and interviewee. You can use focus groups to generate ideas; to explore a variety of different perspectives; or to test potential solutions to problems. Focus groups can be useful to explore sensitive topics, but in this situation a lot of care needs to be taken, especially around group composition and establishing ground rules.

Arranging a time for a focus group that suits all the attendees can be challenging. Ready-made groups, such as a memory café that regularly meets in the library, have the advantage that participants already know one another and are likely to feel comfortable with each other. They are also likely to have a designated time and location that is convenient for members to meet, so you are not asking people to make an additional trip. However, be aware that using an existing group may mean all participants do not meet your ideal selection criteria and, in some cases, may have their own ways of interacting that are not best suited to a focus group discussion. For example, if carers tend to dominate the group, it may be difficult to shift the emphasis towards people with dementia.

Whilst focus groups usually have six to eight participants, a slightly smaller group, with around three to five participants, may work better for people with dementia. Be aware that some people with dementia may find it difficult to follow a group conversation and may need additional support, especially in a larger group. Recapping the discussion so far on a regular basis can be helpful. The room needs to be private and reasonably quiet so the focus group can be conducted without distractions. Acoustics can also be important: a room with a lot of echo can make it difficult to follow the conversation.

As with interviews, the communication tips in Chapter 2 are likely to be useful when facilitating a focus group involving people with dementia. Some additional tools that may help include using post-it notes so that people can write down an idea they want to share whilst someone else is talking, or if they prefer to do that rather than speak. Having someone available to write for participants, if they wish, can be helpful. You can also give each participant a card to hold up to indicate they want to speak.

If some participants are struggling to follow a group conversation, there are a variety of activities you can ask people to do in pairs (and possibly then share with the group). One option is to use a set of flashcards with ideas or options you are interested in, for instance activities that are offered in the library. The cards can contain words and/or images depending on what you feel will be most helpful for the group. You can ask participants to sort these into an order (for example from most to least important), sort them into categories or otherwise arrange the cards to help you better understand their views. Depending on the group, they might also add their own suggestions on blank cards.

Visual methods

Visual methods can be useful when conducting research or evaluation involving people affected by dementia. Discussing dementia can produce strong emotions and images can be a 'safer' medium to express uncomfortable or sensitive thoughts or experiences that are difficult to talk about (especially within an unfamiliar group). For any of us, it can be difficult to express feelings or emotions through words alone and images can sometimes help to convey experiences more effectively or powerfully. Furthermore, the process of producing an image usually allows participants more time to reflect on the topic being explored, which can be helpful to give people with dementia more time to think about their responses rather than being expected to make an immediate verbal response.

Visual methods have the potential to be used to explore a variety of issues in relation to library use, from people's emotions around the way they view the library, to more practical issues such as library design or colour schemes.

Some suggestions for ways to make visual methods more accessible for people with dementia (and also for people who may not feel confident with creative activities generally) include:

- doing activities as a group – this usually feels less pressurised
- suggesting participants work in pairs or small groups so people feel less dependent on their individual skills
- emphasising that it is ideas that are important, not artistic skill (for instance showing examples using stick figures)
- ensuring the group is supported by an artist or volunteer who can help to produce images based on participants' descriptions
- offering options such as photography, collage or manipulating stock images (that is, methods that do not require people to draw).

Another approach that can be useful is to provide more structure to the activity by introducing pre-created images, rather than asking participants to produce their own. This might involve participants ordering or sequencing a series of pre-made images or completing a sequence of images. Alternatively, it might mean adding detail to a basic image, for instance, asking participants to complete empty speech or thought bubbles to suggest what characters are saying and/or thinking.

For some people with dementia, Talking Mats (www.talkingmats.com) may be helpful. Talking Mats are a way to engage with people with communication or cognitive difficulties, including those who have dementia. In essence, they are similar to the card sorting activities described in the focus group section above. Using a Talking Mat, a participant is given a series of options, one at a time, and asked to think about what they feel about each one. They place the symbol on a visual scale to indicate how they feel about it (for example, happy, unhappy, unsure). If a person with dementia has previous experience of using Talking Mats, it may be useful to adopt a similar approach to ask about their experiences of library services.

Ethics

For some research, you will need to gain permission from an ethics committee before you are able to collect data. This might be an external body such as an NHS Research Committee, your own organisation or a funder or partner organisation. Whether or not you need to obtain formal ethical approval, it is good practice to provide your participants with written information about your research or evaluation prior to the activity. This should be written in accessible language for participants and explain:

- exactly what they will be expected to do
- the fact that participation is voluntary and they do not have to answer or do anything they are not comfortable with

- how the results will be used
- how data will be stored securely
- contact details in case of queries or concerns
- confidentiality and anonymity (for example, confirming responses will be anonymised in reports)
- how to withdraw from the research if they wish and any limitations on this.

Providing written information that participants can take away and re-read is important. However, you should also repeat the main points verbally prior to the activity to check they have understood and have an opportunity to ask questions. This is especially important when working with people with dementia. Once they are happy with the ethical issues around the research, participants usually sign a consent form. Alternatively, it is possible to record consent verbally (audio or video) if this is more appropriate. It is important to think of consent as an ongoing process and ensure that participants continue to give their consent throughout the research, especially if data gathering activities take place over an extended period.

To consent to research, a participant needs to be able to understand and process the information necessary to make an informed decision about taking part. This ability should be considered in the context of the specific research – some research projects are easier to understand, and therefore consent to, than others. A crucial concept when conducting research with people with dementia is the fact that capacity to consent is *not* determined by a person's diagnosis or membership of a particular group but is unique to that person. Furthermore, capacity to consent is not static; it can fluctuate over time (Biros, 2018). In practice, for most research activities within a community setting, it is likely that the people with dementia will be able to consent themselves – especially if the research can be explained in a relatively straightforward way. However, you may also wish to ask for assent from a carer or relative if they usually accompany the person with dementia.

A final ethical consideration is the importance of informing people how the insights you gather from their involvement have been used. Providing this in a variety of media can be helpful. This might include a short, simple summary accompanied by 'before' and 'after' photographs or a video demonstrating or discussing the changes made as a result of the research.

Conclusions

Living with dementia is something that can be incredibly difficult for those of us without the condition to imagine and relate to. It is therefore important to involve people with dementia directly in the evaluation and development of library services to ensure that these meet their actual needs, not simply our perceptions of what those needs might be. Involving people with dementia in research and evaluation activities requires a degree of flexibility and adaptation, but many of these considerations are simply good practice and paying attention to them can benefit other participants too.

Research and evaluation are important to plan how to adapt library services to meet the changing needs of people with dementia. The final chapter considers some of the ways in which the demographics of people with dementia and the approaches to their care might be expected to change in the future. Involving people with dementia and their carers in the ongoing development of library services will be crucial to ensure that libraries continue to adapt their provision to best meet the needs of customers affected by dementia.

10
Future Trends

> It's less about a prescribed set of next steps and more about just sharing that vision and working together on what that means . . .
>
> (Abby Wolfe, Public Awareness Co-ordinator,
> Alzheimer Society of Saskatchewan, Canada, in conversation with author)

This chapter shifts from looking at current practice to exploring anticipated trends that are likely to have an impact on the ways in which libraries might support people with dementia and their carers. This includes both changes within populations likely to be diagnosed with dementia and developments in the provision of care. It concludes by suggesting actions libraries may want to consider to ensure the ways in which people with dementia and their carers are supported meet the needs of these customers in the future. This chapter offers a broad overview of issues that may impact on the provision of library services generally; however, for any library, it is important to assess predicted trends in the local population – the factors that are likely to have the greatest impact on provision can vary considerably from region to region.

Demographic changes

The first factor likely to impact on the provision of dementia care and support is the expected increase in the number of people diagnosed with the condition worldwide. The number of people living with dementia around the world is expected to increase substantially over the coming decades. Researchers estimate that the number of people with dementia will increase from 57.4 million cases globally in 2019 to 152.8 million cases in 2050. The largest increases in projected dementia cases are in North Africa and the Middle East

(367%) and eastern sub-Saharan Africa (357%). The smallest percentage changes are anticipated in high-income countries in Asia Pacific and western Europe, where they are expected to rise by 53% and 74% respectively (Nichols et al., 2019). Even in countries where the expected percentage increases are comparatively modest, the numbers are still striking. The number of people with dementia in the UK is forecast to reach over 1 million by 2025 and over 2 million by 2051 (ARUK, 2022). In the US an estimated 7.2 million people are expected to have Alzheimer's disease by 2025; in the absence of medical breakthroughs, the number is expected to climb to 13.8 million by 2060 (Alzheimer's Association, 2021).

Substantial increases in the numbers of people diagnosed with dementia will inevitably mean more pressure on care services and demands for additional provision. In the absence of significant increases in health and social care budgets, this is likely to result in greater demand for community-based support via public, community and charitable services for families affected by dementia – including through libraries. In addition, it is important that provision adapts to different generations likely to be affected by dementia. People who were 70 in 2020 were teenagers in the 1960s so are not likely to be able to relate strongly to VE Day images, for example.

In addition to the increasing number of dementia cases, changes are forecast within specific population groups that are likely to have an impact on the provision of dementia care. Some of the demographic factors that are likely to be most significant in the future include ethnic diversity, LBGT (lesbian, gay, bisexual and transgender) communities and people ageing without children.

Ethnic diversity

The most pressing issues around ethnic diversity and dementia differ in different parts of the world. In the UK, for example, there is an awareness that immigrant communities who arrived in the country in the mid- to late-20th century are now ageing and likely to experience increasing numbers of dementia cases over the coming decades. Elsewhere, for instance in Australasia, there is increasing awareness of the importance of providing dementia services that meet the needs of indigenous communities appropriately. The following section briefly outlines some considerations around support for people from both migrant and indigenous communities whose needs might not be met effectively through current mainstream dementia provision.

Migrant communities

The UK is an example of a country where changes in the demographic profile of migrant communities is likely to have an impact on dementia care over the coming decades. There is little research looking specifically at dementia amongst minority ethnic groups. As a result, there are no exact figures regarding the prevalence of dementia in these groups. In 2013 the number of cases was estimated to be around 25,000 (APPG on Dementia, 2013). However, this figure is predicted to grow to 160,000 by 2051 (Khan, 2015). Furthermore, it is acknowledged that any figure is likely to be a significant underestimate as dementia has been characterised as a 'hidden problem' for many minority ethnic communities (Wilkinson, 2002).

People from minority ethnic communities often receive a diagnosis of dementia at a later stage than those from white communities for a number of reasons. These can include concerns about stigma related to dementia; beliefs that care services are inadequate and families are better placed to care for someone; previous negative experiences of health services; normalisation of memory problems; concern about receiving a diagnosis; and language barriers (Ahmed et al., 2014; Sagbakken et al., 2020). Research has reported a perception that dementia does not affect black people because they are not seen in the media as a population at risk of developing the condition, despite the fact that Black African and Caribbean elders have a higher prevalence and a younger onset of dementia compared with the white UK population (Berwald et al., 2016). There may also be differences in coping strategies employed. For example, Moïse Roche and colleagues found that religiosity was important in understanding and managing dementia as people from Black African and Caribbean communities often drew strength and support in prayer and religion (Roche et al., 2021).

As well as the increasing number of people from minority ethnic communities likely to be diagnosed with dementia, there is evidence that individuals from these backgrounds may also be more likely to be carers. For example, members of the British-Bangladeshi community are three times more likely to be carers than White British populations (Hossain and Khan, 2019). There is also some evidence that members of particular minority ethnic communities may view caring differently. A review of research into perceptions and experiences of dementia found that, amongst Black African and Caribbean groups, carers experienced less emotional burden from caring for relatives with dementia than their white counterparts; they also tended to find more satisfaction in their role (Roche et al., 2021).

Although research into dementia care provision for minority ethnic populations is currently limited, the trends indicated above suggest that libraries in a number of countries and regions will increasingly need to consider how they offer support to people with dementia and their carers from a range of ethnic backgrounds. There are examples of specialist dementia services available for some communities that libraries may be able to learn from; for example, Touchstone's BME (Black and Minority Ethnic) Dementia Service in Leeds in the UK provides culturally appropriate dementia awareness talks in a variety of languages and runs a South Asian Dementia Café (Touchstone, 2022). Another example is Jewish Care (n.d.), which provides care homes, memory cafés, carers' support groups and other services for people with dementia in the south-east of England. It may be possible for libraries to partner with these types of organisations to offer services for specific groups or to draw on their advice and support to ensure activities are inclusive to all communities.

Another resource that libraries might utilise is the skills of their staff and volunteers from various minority ethnic communities. Having staff who speak community languages or have first-hand knowledge of cultural activities in different communities can often be helpful when making connections with people with dementia from a range of backgrounds. However, it is important to avoid making assumptions based on ethnicity or cultural background; for instance, not assuming that people from ostensibly similar backgrounds will automatically have a connection – what is sometimes called 'identity matching'.

Likely changes in the ethnic composition of populations living with dementia mean libraries will need to rethink the types of resources they provide, as well as services offered. Whilst there are examples of organisations that design resources for people with dementia from particular minority ethnic communities, the availability of published resources can be quite limited. The Black Dementia Company (2022) is one example; it publishes resources based on familiarity with African and Caribbean cultures. Their product range includes puzzles, colouring books and other activity books that are intended to be used as part of social engagement with people living with dementia. When considering resources that meet the needs of minority ethnic communities, translation is also likely to be necessary in some instances. However, it is important to be mindful of the complexities around the translation of materials about dementia, as discussed in Chapter 8.

Indigenous communities

Whilst the provision of support for migrant communities is a key issue in many countries, in some regions, how to best serve members of indigenous populations living with dementia is also a crucial concern. For many indigenous communities, formal medical care is often not viewed as the only way to support people with dementia. Other techniques such as prayer, ceremony, church, meditation, yoga, visiting with youth, art-therapy, storytelling, speaking the language and using humour can be equally important (I-CAARE, 2017).

An example of how the information needs of indigenous peoples might be met is the Caring for Spirit website for Aboriginal and Torres Strait Islander communities in Australia (https://caringforspirit.neura.edu.au). Dementia rates are three to five times higher in these communities than the broader Australian population. This website aims to provide a centralised online source of appropriate resources and information for Aboriginal and Torres Strait Islander communities by translating the results of current research into culturally relevant and accessible information, education and training for people living with dementia, their families and carers, and Aboriginal and Torres Strait Islander health workers. The website includes videos of people from Aboriginal and Torres Strait Islander communities talking about dementia. It uses language designed to resonate with the target audience and draws on ways of thinking about the world within these communities (NeuRA, 2019).

As with migrant communities, staff or volunteers who are members of indigenous communities can be helpful in making connections between the library and these communities, but it is important that working with indigenous communities is seen as something that *everyone* should engage in, not only those staff who share a common background. Abby Wolfe from the Alzheimer Society of Saskatchewan in Canada describes her approach to working with indigenous communities with whom she does not share a cultural background, in particular the importance of supporting communities to generate their own responses and actions that are meaningful for them:

> We have a large First Nations population in Saskatchewan and some areas are set up as First Nations reserves. So, we have had experience of being invited onto reserves to do presentations for their community groups. Often, it's at a health centre or as part of their community health day, and those have been very important opportunities for us to build those relationships and ensure that we are helping to grow connections in those communities. The consideration that is always at the forefront of my mind when I do those presentations is how do I approach it with cultural humility and how do I approach it in a way that recognises that they may have some different perspectives about what dementia means? It's maybe not my role to lead or describe next steps. It really has to be generated from what are they identifying they want from us and how we can facilitate that in the best way. As much as we can, we want the community that we're working with to feel like they have the ownership of their dementia-

friendly progress: they're identifying the vision and then they're moving towards that in a way that is meaningful for them. So, I think that aligns really well with being able to build relationships with First Nations communities and to respect that need for their autonomy or leadership efforts.

(A. Wolfe, conversation with author, 15 November 2021)

LGBT+ communities

LGBT+ communities are another group who are likely to form a larger segment of the population affected by dementia in the future. However, identifying people with dementia who are from this community is far from straightforward. The number of people with dementia who are LGBT+ is likely to be significantly underestimated at present and this is likely to be an increasingly important group for libraries to consider in terms of dementia-friendly service provision in the future.

Research has shown that LGBT+ older adults are more likely to exhibit particular vulnerabilities that can exacerbate the challenges of living well with dementia, such as disproportionately high levels of social isolation and stigmatisation as they age. According to a US survey in 2014, one-third of LGBT+ older people reported living alone and 40% said that their support networks had become smaller over time (Espinoza, 2014). The issues faced by an LGBT+ person with dementia can be complex. For example, their carer may be someone who is not supportive of their identity. Also, dementia may bring back older memories, so some LGBT+ people may sometimes feel that they are in a time before they came out and this might bring distressing emotions. They may also recall memories from the past when they experienced prejudice, discrimination and harassment.

LGBT+ carers also face challenges. Research in the US reports that LGBT+ people become carers at a higher rate than the general population (one in five compared to one in six) (AARP and National Alliance for Caregiving, 2015). Adult children who are LGBT+ and do not have children of their own may be expected to care for a parent. However, LGBT+ people may not be 'out' to the person they are caring for or may be caring for someone who does not accept, or does not remember, their identity, relationship or gender expression.

When designing publicity materials or writing descriptions for dementia-friendly events and services, it is important to ensure these are inclusive of LGBT+ people with dementia and their carers, for example, in terms of the language and images used. To make sure LGBT+ people feel welcome at all activities, it is worth thinking about the assumptions that might be made about families, lifestyles and life experiences. For instance, when planning questions for a reminiscence session, try to make sure the themes to be discussed are something everyone will be able to relate to. It may also be worth considering setting up an LGBT+-specific memory café or support group, perhaps in collaboration with a local LGBT+ support organisation.

As well as offering services for LGBT+ people with dementia and their carers, libraries can be ideal venues for events to increase awareness of the older LGBT+ community, including those with dementia, within the wider community. The Silver Pride event at Belong Crewe care home, where my dad lived, is held annually to coincide with Pride Month and is an example of the type of activity that might work well in a library. This event is run in association with partners including a local sexual health charity and older people's LGBT+ network. The event is usually open to the local community, as well as staff and residents. Activities have included musical performances and open mic acts; craft activities, such as making rainbow suncatchers; opportunities for people to reminisce prompted by displays of artefacts from the history of the LGBT+ movement; and the provision of information about practical and emotional support available locally for members of the LGBT+ community.

People ageing without children

Another demographic trend that is likely to have implications for dementia care in some countries is the increasing number of older people who do not have children or whose children live too far away to care for them on a day-to-day basis. In the UK it is estimated that the number of people over 65 without adult children will rise to 2 million by 2030. Whilst only 9% of women born in the 1940s have not become mothers, it is estimated that 25% of those born in the 1970s will not do so. Figures on fathers are not recorded in the same way, but it is estimated that 23% of men over 45 are without children. Within some communities, the numbers are considerably higher: 90% of LGBT+ people and 85% of people with disabilities are estimated to be ageing without children (Ageing Without Children, 2021).

People with dementia who do not have children can be particularly vulnerable as they may lack someone to advocate on their behalf. This obviously has implications for the health and social care sector as people without children often move into residential care earlier. However, it also has implications for community organisations such as libraries. For example, people with dementia may need additional support from library staff or volunteers to attend activities or to use the library if they do not have someone available to attend with them.

Changes in care provision

As well as demographic changes that are likely to impact on support for people with dementia and their carers, there are also likely to be changes to the way that care is provided in the future. This may include changes to care models, the use of technology and the long-term impacts of the COVID-19 pandemic.

Care models

An important factor that could affect the ways in which libraries support people with dementia and their carers is an increasing emphasis in a number of countries on community-based care and 'ageing in place' (Pani-Harreman et al., 2021). According to a report into new models of home care in the UK, a key theme is a 'focus on wellbeing, prevention, promoting independence and connection to communities – to be able to stay in their own homes and be supported to do things themselves. This may include linking people to be able to contribute to their local communities and social groups' (Bennett et al., 2018, 6).

An example of how this can work in practice is local area co-ordination, an approach that began in Australia to support people with learning disabilities and has since been adopted in a number of countries and for a range of service users. It operates a single point of contact and builds relationships with individuals, families and communities to develop networks of stakeholders, allowing co-ordinators or 'community navigators' to draw support from the community. This enables individuals to maximise their independence and connections to their communities. The local area co-ordination approach recognises that people's needs often go beyond the physical. It focuses on local relationships and assistance and aims to add value to existing support services, rather than replacing them (Bennett et al., 2018).

An alternative model that performs a similar role is community circles, which informally co-ordinate support from friends, family and neighbours. These can put people in touch with things that may have an impact on their wellbeing but are not necessarily within the remit of health or social care services – for example, putting them in touch with a bowling club or a faith community to prevent loneliness. Community circles go beyond signposting; they support the person to maximise their independence and involvement (Bennett et al., 2018).

It is easy to envisage how libraries might play a crucial role in initiatives such as local area co-ordination or community circles. Library services have the potential to become key players in stakeholder networks through building relationships that can support people's community connections and emotional needs.

Developments in technology

Developments in technology are also likely to have an impact on care for people with dementia and on the ways in which libraries might support them. Virtual reality (VR), for example, can be used as part of reminiscence activities or to provide relaxation experiences. At present, this usually occurs on a small scale or as part of research projects (for example, Appel et al., 2021), but if these pilots prove successful it could well become more widespread and libraries could have a role in facilitating wider access to these types of emerging technologies.

Impact of COVID-19

At the time of writing this book in mid-2022, the long-term effects of the COVID-19 pandemic are still unknown. However, there are a number of potential impacts that may have implications for the ways in which libraries support people with dementia and their carers over the next few years. Many of the public health measures introduced to try to limit the spread of COVID-19 have been particularly difficult for people with dementia. Engaging with people through a range of senses is an important feature of dementia care. Measures such as social distancing, limitations on the number of people in certain spaces and mask wearing inevitably limited opportunities for the use of different senses and restricted communal activities such as singing, as well as potentially exacerbating the communication difficulties that many people with dementia experience.

From March 2020 many of the services offered to people with dementia were paused for more than two years and in some cases it is not yet certain when, or if, they will be reintroduced. For many people, and in particular people with dementia, the pandemic increased isolation and the full effects of this are not yet known. It may be that some people are keen to return to face-to-face activities as soon as possible, but others may be fearful after such an extended period of isolation. In some cases, while it has not been possible to continue to run face-to-face activities, libraries have offered an increased range of remote services. As was discussed in Chapter 6, although online activities can be successful in the right circumstances, there are significant challenges in offering a full range of services online in the longer term.

Chapter 7 discussed some of the difficulties libraries frequently face when working with care homes and these challenges inevitably increased as care homes were, effectively, cut off from communities. Again, at the time of writing, whilst many restrictions have been relaxed, it is unknown how long some measures might continue to protect people in care homes and what effective models of partnership working with this sector might look like in the future.

Conclusion: future library provision for people with dementia and their carers

Demand for dementia-friendly library services is only likely to increase in the future as the numbers of people affected by dementia rise and there is greater emphasis on community-based care. However, the types of provision offered cannot be static; libraries will need to continually adapt in line with changes in the demographic profile of people with dementia in different localities.

It is clear that libraries have enormous potential to support people with dementia and their carers, but in many cases this potential is not being fully realised at present. This can be true even in libraries that have been specifically designed to be dementia friendly because, as discussed in Chapter 3, the way that they operate on a day-to-day basis often means they are not as accessible for people with dementia as they could easily be. Staff knowledge and understanding are crucial. Naturally, library staff cannot be expected to be experts in dementia care, but a basic understanding of what makes for a dementia-friendly environment and service can potentially make a huge difference to someone's experience of their library. Partnership working with organisations that have expertise in dementia care is vital to ensure library provision is inclusive. Reflecting this inclusivity in messaging and publicity is important, but it is vital that dementia-friendly messaging is backed up by practice. The best way to ensure this is the case is to involve people with dementia and their carers in any service reviews or evaluations to discover first-hand whether library services are meeting their needs.

Taking action to create a dementia-friendly library can feel initially like a massive undertaking, but small changes can make a big difference. Whilst not every library can have a full refurbishment, any library can take simple measures such as decluttering noticeboards, making sure entrances are clear and welcoming and ensuring publicity materials use dementia-positive language and images.

In efforts to make libraries more dementia friendly, no single library or individual has all the answers and there is immense value in sharing experiences and learning from each other, particularly within a locality or library sector. As Abby Wolfe from the Alzheimer Society of Saskatchewan in Canada explains, seeing an example they can directly relate to often helps people to see how dementia friendliness can work in practice for them:

> When I talk about the global literature around dementia friendliness, it's almost like it's too grand or too ambiguous for them to really latch on to. But the more that I can talk about local examples, or really share how folks in a closer geographic area have done things, that's actually what seems to do the trick.
>
> (A. Wolfe, conversation with author, 15 November 2021)

When providing activities, programmes and services within the library, options specifically aimed at people with dementia are likely to be necessary in some cases. In other instances, it is worth thinking about how to ensure people with dementia feel included in mainstream provision, perhaps by providing extra support.

Technology has a role to play in library provision of course, but it is not a solution on its own. One of the positive outcomes of the COVID-19 pandemic is that it stimulated the introduction of new online forms of provision that may not have seemed feasible in the past. The challenge of the next few years will be to research and test these new possibilities so that technology is used in the best ways possible to meet the needs of people with dementia and their carers.

One of the strengths of libraries is that they can offer a space where people with dementia and their carers can share experiences. Examples described in previous chapters, such as Scottish Book Trust's Reading is Caring and Sefton Libraries' Lost Voices project, demonstrate that libraries can design activities in ways that offer something for both the person with dementia and the person caring for them. Both can get something out of taking part in an activity and enjoy spending time together. This can be particularly true for creative or imaginative activities that allow for more of a level playing field in comparison to activities that rely on skills such as memory or verbal communication.

Activities for people with dementia that emphasise the role of imagination, rather than memory, draw on the unique feature of libraries as cultural organisations that promote books and other resources to foster imagination and escapism. Whilst it makes sense for organisations such as museums and archives to offer reminiscence resources, for galleries to support visual arts and theatres to promote performing arts, libraries' distinctive strength lies in helping people with dementia to enjoy and share imaginative responses and ideas. Of course, libraries can be fantastic venues for other activities too, particularly in collaboration with partners. However, it is in creating opportunities for imagination through reading books – and also other types of 'texts' – that libraries can, perhaps, make their greatest contribution to dementia care. At present this notion is underdeveloped, in both research and practice, but hopefully it is a possibility that will be explored further in the future.

Finally, when working with people with dementia, there can be a tendency to stick to topics or activities that are considered 'nice' or 'safe'. Obviously, it is important to be aware of the implications of introducing certain subjects and consider how people may be affected. However, this does not mean having to avoid more complex, challenging or controversial issues completely. An example is the Silver Pride event mentioned above, which may open up the possibility of challenging discussions or responses. This tendency to stick to safe options is also often seen in the choices of literature, music or other resources offered to groups or individuals with dementia – or indeed to older people more generally. As a facilitator in the Words in Mind bibliotherapy project (see Chapter 4) commented, texts selected for groups of people with mental health issues tended to be 'more edgy' than those chosen for people with dementia. Whilst more challenging choices will not be suitable for everyone, they should not be automatically excluded from consideration when working with people with dementia.

Summary: ten actions for dementia-friendly libraries

Ensuring your library is dementia friendly can feel like an enormous task, especially if you are located in a poorly designed building and have limited time and resources. This book therefore concludes by describing ten relatively simple steps that libraries can take to ensure their services and environments cater for the needs of people with dementia and their carers. Exactly how each suggested action is implemented will vary from library to library, depending on its customer base, resources, local partnership possibilities and a range of other factors. Naturally, it is not necessary to do everything at once; in fact, it is better to take small steps and then ask for feedback from customers affected by dementia on ways to improve further.

1. Support *all* library staff to gain a basic understanding of dementia and how they can best support customers, colleagues and other members of the community who may have dementia or are caring for someone with the condition. This includes staff such as caretakers and cleaners who may interact with customers with dementia within their role and are likely to be responsible for tasks such as arranging furniture. (See Chapter 2 for examples of training provision.)
2. Explore ways to involve customers living with dementia and their carers in decisions about service development. This could initially be on an informal basis; for example, simply chatting to them about how easily they can find their way around the library, borrow resources, etc. (See Chapter 9 for more suggestions of consultation methods.)
3. Find out where there are gaps in provision locally. Making sure information on local services is up to date means that libraries can effectively signpost customers to relevant services and allows library staff to consider where they might be able to help fill gaps, perhaps in

partnership with other organisations. (See Chapters 4 and 5 for examples of the types of services and activities libraries might offer.)

4. Develop partnerships with a range of organisations to raise awareness of the ways in which the library can offer support for people with dementia and their carers and to explore ways of working collaboratively to improve services. (See Chapter 7 for advice on working in partnership.)
5. Consider simple ways in which the library environment can be made more dementia friendly; for example, decluttering entrance areas and noticeboards. (See Chapter 3 for more ideas.)
6. Consider what resources the library has that may be helpful for people with dementia. This can include titles specifically for people with dementia, but also general resources that could be curated by the library. For example, packaging together poetry and image books on a common theme along with ideas for questions for a carer and person with dementia to discuss. Think about how customers will go about finding these resources (for example, are they labelled in some way, shelved in a separate section or highlighted in the catalogue?). (See Chapter 4 for examples.)
7. Explore whether there is demand for online provision to reach more people affected by dementia, especially those who live further from the library. If so, what types of support are needed? Are there opportunities to work in partnership, for example, with the library offering technical support and advice to help people with dementia or their carers join online activities run by another organisation? (See Chapter 6 for examples.)
8. Review publicity and communications materials to ensure these are dementia friendly in terms of language and design. (See Chapter 8 for details.)
9. Consider how the library supports staff, volunteers and colleagues affected by dementia. What additional support might be offered to people diagnosed with dementia or caring for someone with the condition? (See Chapter 2 for suggestions.)
10. Share experiences of dementia-friendly library provision through networking within the library sector and beyond. There is still a lot we do not know about dementia, so sharing examples of what works in libraries from different sectors and locations is crucial.

References

AARP and National Alliance for Caregiving (2015) *Caregiving in the US*, AARP, www.aarp.org/content/dam/aarp/ppi/2015/caregiving-in-the-united-states-2015-report-revised.pdf

Aged Care Quality and Safety Commission (2021) *Aged Care Quality Standards*, Australian Government, www.agedcarequality.gov.au/sites/default/files/media/acqsc_aged_care_quality_standards_fact_sheet_4pp_v8.pdf

Ageing Without Children (2021) Statistics, www.awwoc.org/statistics

Ahmed, A., Yates-Bolton, N. J., and Collier, E. H. (2014) *Diversity and Inclusiveness in Dementia: Listening Event Report*, Salford Institute for Dementia, http://usir.salford.ac.uk/id/eprint/35270

Akron-Summit County Public Library (2022) *Your Dementia-inclusive Library*, www.akronlibrary.org/about/accessibility/dementia-inclusive

All Party Parliamentary Group (APPG) on Dementia (2013) *Dementia Does Not Discriminate: The Experiences of Black, Asian and Minority Ethnic Communities*, APPG on Dementia, www.alzheimers.org.uk/sites/default/files/migrate/downloads/appg_2013_bame_report.pdf

All Party Parliamentary Group (APPG) on Arts, Health and Wellbeing (2017) *Creative Health: The Arts for Health and Wellbeing*, APPG, www.artshealthresources.org.uk/docs/creative-health-the-arts-for-health-and-wellbeing

All Party Parliamentary Group (APPG) on Dementia (2019) *Hidden No More: Dementia and Disability*, Alzheimer's Society, www.alzheimers.org.uk/sites/default/files/2019-06/APPG_on_Dementia_2019_report_Hidden_no_more_dementia_and_disability_media.pdf

Alzheimer Society of Canada (2017) *2017 Awareness Survey: Executive Summary*, Alzheimer Society of Canada, https://alzheimer.ca/sites/default/files/documents/2017_AWARENESS-SURVEY_EXECUTIVE_SUMMARY_0.pdf

Alzheimer Society of Canada (2022) *Dementia-Friendly Canada*, https://alzheimer.ca/en/take-action/become-dementia-friendly/dementia-friendly-canada

Alzheimer Society of Saskatchewan (2019) *Dementia Friendly Toolkit: The Library Edition*, Alzheimer Society of Saskatchewan.

Alzheimer's Association (2021) Alzheimer's Disease Facts and Figures, *Alzheimer's & Dementia*, **202**, 327–406.

Alzheimer's Association (2022) *Parkinson's Disease Dementia*, www.alz.org/alzheimers-dementia/what-is-dementia/types-of-dementia/parkinson-s-disease-dementia

Alzheimer's Disease International (ADI) (2016) *Dementia Friendly Communities: Key Principles*, ADI, www.alzint.org/u/dfc-principles.pdf

Alzheimer's Research UK (ARUK) (2015) *Women and Dementia: A Marginalised Majority*, ARUK, www.alzheimersresearchuk.org/wp-content/uploads/2015/03/Women-and-Dementia-A-Marginalised-Majority1.pdf

Alzheimer's Research UK (ARUK) (2022) *Statistics about Dementia – Dementia Statistics Hub*, www.dementiastatistics.org/statistics-about-dementia

Alzheimer's Society (2014) *Dementia 2014: Opportunity for Change*, Alzheimer's Society.

Alzheimer's Society (2015a) *How to Help People with Dementia: A Guide for Customer-facing Staff*, Alzheimer's Society.

Alzheimer's Society (2015b) *Creating a Dementia-friendly Workplace: A Practical Guide for Employers*, Alzheimer's Society.

Alzheimer's Society (2016) *Over Half of People Fear Dementia Diagnosis*, last modified 13 May, www.alzheimers.org.uk/news/2018-05-29/over-half-people-fear-dementia-diagnosis-62-cent-think-it-means-life-over

Alzheimer's Society (2017a) *What is Alzheimer's Disease? Factsheet 401LP*, Alzheimer's Society, www.alzheimers.org.uk/sites/default/files/2019-09/What%20is%20Alzheimer%27s%20disease.pdf

Alzheimer's Society (2017b) *Dementia Friends*, www.dementiafriends.org.uk

Alzheimer's Society (2018) *Positive Language: An Alzheimer's Society Guide to Talking about Dementia*, Alzheimer's Society, www.alzheimers.org.uk/sites/default/files/2018-09/Positive%20language%20guide_0.pdf

Alzheimer's Society (2019a) *What is Mild Cognitive Impairment (MCI)? Factsheet 470LP*, Alzheimer's Society, www.alzheimers.org.uk/sites/default/files/2019-09/470lp-what-is-mild-cognitive-impairment-mci-190521.pdf

REFERENCES

Alzheimer's Society (2020) *The Impact of COVID-19 on People Affected by Dementia*, Alzheimer's Society, www.alzheimers.org.uk/sites/default/files/2020-08/The_Impact_of_COVID-19_on_People_Affected_By_Dementia.pdf

Alzheimer's Society (2021) How Many People Have Dementia in the UK? *Alzheimer's Society Blog*, December 13, www.alzheimers.org.uk/blog/how-many-people-have-dementia-uk

Alzheimer's Society (2022) *What is Vascular Dementia? Factsheet 402LP*, Alzheimer's Society, www.alzheimers.org.uk/sites/default/files/2022-05/402LP-what-is-vascular-dementia.pdf

American Library Association (ALA) (2020) *Library Services for Patrons with Alzheimer's/Dementia*, www.ala.org/advocacy/diversity/services-alzheimers

Appel, L., Ali, S., Narag, T., Mozeson, K., Pasat, Z., Orchanian-Cheff, A., Campos, J. L. (2021) Virtual Reality to Promote Wellbeing in Persons with Dementia: A Scoping Review, *Journal of Rehabilitation and Assistive Technologies Engineering*, January 2021.

Australian Institute of Health and Welfare (AIHW) (2021) *Dementia in Australia 2021: Summary Report*, AIHW, www.aihw.gov.au/getmedia/13eeb292-dc65-445c-9ba0-874ef2f54996/aihw-dem-3.pdf

Bamford, S. M., Holley-Moore, J. and Watson, J. A. (2014) *Compendium of Essays: New Perspectives and Approaches to Understanding Dementia and Stigma*, ILC-UK.

Batsch, N. L. and Mittelman, M. S. (2012) *World Alzheimer Report 2012: Overcoming the Stigma of Dementia*, Alzheimer's Disease International, www.alzint.org/u/WorldAlzheimerReport2012.pdf

Bedford Free Public Library (2022) *Doll for Dementia Patients*, www.bedfordlibrary.net/resources/library-of-things/doll-for-dementia-patients

Behuniak, S. M. (2011) The Living Dead? The Construction of People with Alzheimer's Disease as Zombies, *Ageing and Society*, **3** (1), 70–92.

Bennett, L., Honeyman, M. and Bottery, S. (2018) *New Models of Home Care*, The King's Fund, www.kingsfund.org.uk/sites/default/files/2018-12/New-models-of-home-care.pdf

Berwald, S., Roche, M., Adelman, S., Mukadam, N. and Livingston, G. (2016) Black African and Caribbean British Communities' Perceptions of Memory Problems: 'We Don't Do Dementia', *PLoS One*, **11** (4), e0151878.

Billington, J., Carroll, J., Davis, P., Healey, C. and Kinderman, P. (2013) A Literature-based Intervention for Older People Living with Dementia, *Perspectives in Public Health*, **133** (3), 165–73.

Biros, M. (2018) Capacity, Vulnerability, and Informed Consent for Research, *The Journal of Law, Medicine and Ethics*, **46** (1), 72–8.

Black Dementia Company (2022) *Created Specially for You!*, www.theblackdementiacompany.com

Bluecoat (n.d.) *Where the Arts Belong*, www.thebluecoat.org.uk/projects/where-the-arts-belong

BookTrust (2019) *Books on Dementia*, www.booktrust.org.uk/booklists/c/childrens-books-on-dementia

Bould, E. (2018) *Dementia-friendly Media and Broadcast Guide*, Alzheimer's Society.

Bracken, G. (2020) Reading Interest: A Book Club That's Raising Self-esteem, *Dementia Together Magazine*, Feb/Mar, www.alzheimers.org.uk/dementia-together-magazine-febmar-20/reading-interest-book-club-thats-raising-self-esteem

Brewster, E. A. (2011) An Investigation of Experiences of Reading for Mental Health and Well-being and Their Relation to Models of Bibliotherapy, PhD, University of Sheffield.

Brewster, L. (2017) Murder by the Book: Using Crime Fiction as a Bibliotherapeutic Resource, *Medical Humanities*, **43**, 62–7.

Brewster, L. and McNicol, S. (2019) *Words in Mind: Evaluation Report*, Lancaster University, https://figshare.com/articles/book/WiM_-_report_-_final_docx/14730771/1

Brewster, L. and McNicol, S. (2021) Bibliotherapy in Practice: A Person-centred Approach to Using Books for Mental Health and Dementia in the Community, *Medical Humanities*, **47** (4), e12.

British Association for Counselling and Psychotherapy (BACP) (2019) Written Evidence from The British Association for Counselling and Psychotherapy, http://data.parliament.uk/writtenevidence/committeeevidence.svc/evidencedocument/justice-committee/ageing-prison-population/written/105870.html#_ftn17

Brooker, D. (2004) What is Person-centred Care for People with Dementia?, *Reviews in Clinical Gerontology*, **13** (3), 215–22.

Brooker, D. (2007) *Person-centred Dementia Care*, Jessica Kingsley Publishers.

Campaign for Level Boarding (n.d.) *Level Boarding: Building a Safe, Efficient, and Modern Railway*, www.levelboarding.org.uk

Canevelli, M., Valletta, M., Toccaceli Blasi, M., Remoli, G., Sarti, G., Nuti, F. et al. (2020) Facing Dementia During the COVID-19 Outbreak, *Journal of the American Geriatrics Society*, **68** (8), 1673–76.

Carers UK/Employers for Carers (EfC) (2014) *Supporting Employees Who are Caring for Someone with Dementia*, Carers UK.

Casey, A.-N. (2019) Does Social Interaction Reduce Risk of Dementia?, *Blog: The Brain Dialogues, (Centre for Healthy Brain Ageing)*, 1 May, https://cheba.unsw.edu.au/blog/does-social-interaction-reduce-risk-dementia

Clarke, L. (2022) Dementia-friendly Services Open at Wakefield District Libraries, *Wakefield Express*, 19 May, www.wakefieldexpress.co.uk/news/people/dementia-friendly-services-open-at-wakefield-district-libraries-3700213

Cohen, G., Russo, M. J., Campos, J. A. and Allegri, R. F. (2020) Living with Dementia: Increased Level of Caregiver Stress in Times of COVID-19, *International Psychogeriatrics*, **32** (11), 1377–81.

Cohen, L. J. (1992) *Bibliotherapy: The Experience of Therapeutic Reading from the Perspective of the Adult Reader*, University of New York.

Comas-Herrera, A. and Knapp, M. (2016) *Cognitive Stimulation Therapy*, MODEM, https://toolkit.modem-dementia.org.uk/wp-content/uploads/2016/04/CST-Intervention-Summary.pdf

Cowl, A. L. and Gaugler, J. E. (2014) Efficacy of Creative Arts Therapy in Treatment of Alzheimer's Disease and Dementia: A Systematic Literature Review, *Activities, Adaptation & Aging,* **38** (4), 281–330.

Culture Perth & Kinross (2016) *Libraries for Health and Well-being*, www.culturepk.org.uk/libraries/find-health

Dallas Public Library (2018) *Stress Busters Class for Caregivers*, https://dallaslibrary.librarymarket.com/index.php/events/stress-busters-class-caregivers

Dementia Action Alliance (DAA) (2010) *National Dementia Declaration for England*, DAA, www.dementiaaction.org.uk/assets/0001/1915/National_Dementia_Declaration_for_England.pdf

Dementia Action Alliance (DAA) (2017) *Review of the Dementia Statements Companion Paper*, DAA, www.dementiaaction.org.uk/assets/0003/3965/Companion_document_August_2017_branded_final.pdf

Dementia Action Alliance (DAA) (2022) *Local DAAs*, www.dementiaaction.org.uk/local_alliances

Dementia Action Alliance (DAA) (n.d.) *The Stirling Standards for Dementia-friendly Design*, DAA, www.dementiaaction.org.uk/assets/0000/7618/dsdcthe_stirling_standards_for_dementia_120430_1.pdf

Dementia Australia (2021a) *Discrimination and Dementia – Enough is Enough*, Dementia Australia, www.dementia.org.au/sites/default/files/2021-09/DAW-2021-Enough-is-enough-report.pdf

Dementia Australia (2021b) *Dementia Language Guidelines*, Dementia Australia, www.dementia.org.au/sites/default/files/resources/dementia-language-guidelines.pdf

Dementia Engagement and Empowerment Project (DEEP) (2013) *Choosing a Dementia-friendly Meeting Space*, DEEP, http://dementiavoices.org.uk/wp-content/uploads/2013/11/DEEP-Guide-Choosing-a-meeting-space.pdf

Dementia Services Development Centre (DSDC) (2021) *Dementia Friendly Design Tool*, Kirklees Council/DSDC.

Dementia UK (2020) *Using Dolls in Dementia Care (Doll Therapy)*, www.dementiauk.org/get-support/living-with-dementia/doll-therapy

Dementia UK (2022a) *Lewy Body Dementia*, www.dementiauk.org/about-dementia/types-of-dementia/dementia-with-lewy-bodies

Dementia UK (2022b) *Young Onset Dementia Facts and Figures*, www.dementiauk.org/about-dementia/young-onset-dementia/about-young-onset-dementia/facts-and-figures

Derwent Valley Mills (n.d.) *About the Derwent Valley Mills*, www.derwentvalleymills.org/about-the-derwent-valley-mills

Devetach, L. (2010) *La Construcción del Camino Lector*, Comunicarte.

DeVries, D., Bollin, A., Brouwer, K., Marion, A., Nass, H. and Pompilius, A. (2019) The Impact of Reading Groups on Engagement and Social Interaction for Older Adults with Dementia: A Literature Review, *Therapeutic Recreation Journal*, **53** (1), 53–75.

Dovetale Press (2016) *Welcome to Dovetale Press*, www.dovetalepress.com

Dowrick, C., Billington, J., Robinson, J., Hamer, A. and Williams, C. (2012) Get into Reading as an Intervention for Common Mental Health Problems: Exploring Catalysts for Change, *Medical Humanities*, **38** (1), 15–20.

East Cheshire NHS Trust Library & Knowledge Service (2021) *Dementia Knowledge Hub*, www.eastcheshirenhslibrary.net/dementia.html

El Haj, M., Altintas, E., Chapelet, G., Kapogiannis, D. and Gallouj, K. (2020) High Depression and Anxiety in People with Alzheimer's Disease Living in Retirement Homes During the COVID-19 Crisis, *Psychiatry Research*, **291**, 113294.

Elliot, G. (2020) *1970s – The Pivot of Change: Carry On Reading*, DementiAbility Enterprises Inc.

Espinoza, R. (2014) *Out and Visible: The Experiences and Attitudes of Lesbian, Gay, Bisexual and Transgender Older Adults, Ages 45–75*, Services and Advocacy for GLBT Elders, SAGE, www.sageusa.org/wp-content/uploads/2018/05/sageusa-out-visible-lgbt-market-research-full-report.pdf

Forsyth, K., Heathcote, L., Senior, J., Malik, B., Meacock, R., Perryman K. et al. (2020) Dementia and Mild Cognitive Impairment in Prisoners Aged Over 50 Years in England and Wales: A Mixed-methods Study, *Health Services Delivery Research*, **8**, 27.

Genova, L. (2012) *Still Alice*, Simon and Schuster.

Goffman, E. (1963) *Stigma: Notes on the Management of Spoiled Identity*, Prentice Hall.

Granada (2019) 'Calm Corner' Opened at Crewe Station for Those with Hidden Disabilities, *Granada*, 20 June 20, www.itv.com/news/granada/2019-06-20/calm-corner-opened-at-crewe-station-for-those-with-hidden-disabilities

Green, G. and Lakey, L. (2013) *Building Dementia Friendly Communities: A Priority for Everyone*, Alzheimer's Society.

Healey, E. (2015) *Elizabeth is Missing*, Penguin.

HealthyBooks (2022) *Dementia*, www.healthybooks.uk/category/119

Hossain, M. Z. and Khan, H. T. A. (2019) Dementia in the Bangladeshi Diaspora in England: A Qualitative Study of the Myths and Stigmas about Dementia, *Journal of Evaluation in Clinical Practice*, **25** (5), 769–78.

House of Commons Justice Committee (2020) *Ageing Prison Population: Fifth Report of Session 2019–21*, House of Commons, https://committees.parliament.uk/publications/2149/documents/19996/default

Hyde, A., Robertson, M., Houston, A., McKillop, J., Sinclair, M., Larkin, A. and Vaughan, P. (2019) *Drawing from Our Experience: Stories of Travelling with Dementia*, UniVerse, Go Upstream and University of Dundee.

Indigenous Cognition & Aging Awareness Research Exchange (I-CAARE) (2017) *What to Expect After a Diagnosis of Dementia: An Indigenous Persons' Guide*, I-CAARE, https://141419f0-5602-433d-85d2-4d5a8ecfd5ec.filesusr.com/ugd/27ba04_63357f59e3584b1da17ed8e3e5ec95d3.pdf

Inspire (2022) *Community Film Screenings*, www.inspireculture.org.uk/arts-culture/community-film-screenings

International Federation of Library Associations and Institutions (IFLA) (2007) Guidelines for Library Services to Persons with Dementia, *IFLA Professional Reports*, 104, www.ifla.org/wp-content/uploads/2019/05/assets/hq/publications/professional-report/104.pdf

Jacklin, K., Pitawanakwat, K., Blind, M., Jones, L., Otowadjiwan, J., Rowe, R. et al. (2018) *Guidelines to P.I.E.C.E.S. of my Relationships*, Indigenous Cognition and Aging Awareness Research Exchange (I-CAARE) and North East Behavioural Supports Ontario, www.i-caare.ca/_files/ugd/882075_b1e4302b0c294238a3354c855fdd6ef8.pdf

Jewish Care (n.d.) *How We Can Help You*, www.jewishcare.org/how-we-can-help-you

Jopling, K. (2017) Promising Approaches to Living Well with Dementia, Age UK, www.ageuk.org.uk/globalassets/age-uk/documents/reports-and-publications/reports-and-briefings/health—wellbeing/rb_feb2018_promising_approaches_to_living_well_with_dementia_report.pdf

Katzman R. (1976) The Prevalence and Malignancy of Alzheimer Disease: A Major Killer, *Archives of Neurology*, **33** (4), 217–18.

Khan, O. (2015) Dementia and Ethnic Diversity: Numbers and Trends. In Botsford, J. and Harrison Dening, K. (eds), *Dementia, Culture and Ethnicity: Issues for All*, Jessica Kingsley, 21–34.

Kim, C., Wu, B., Tanaka, E., Watanabe, T., Watanabe, K., Chen, W. et al. (2016) Association Between a Change in Social Interaction and Dementia among Elderly People, *International Journal of Gerontology*, **10** (2), 76–80.

Kitwood, T. (1997) *Dementia Reconsidered: The Person Comes First*, Open University Press.

Lancashire County Council (2022) *Kinsgfold Library*, www.lancashire.gov.uk/libraries-and-archives/libraries/find-a-library/kingsfold-library

Leavitt, S. (2012) *Tangles: A Story about Alzheimer's, My Mother, and Me*, Skyhorse Publishing.

Lee, S., O'Neill, D. and Moss, H. (2021) Dementia-inclusive Group Singing Online During COVID-19: A Qualitative Exploration, *Nordic Journal of Music Therapy*, **31** (4), 308–26.

Lewis, J., Enticknap, A. and Poole, G. (2019), Culture Hive Case Study, HST, https://humanstorytheatre.com/wp-content/uploads/2020/06/Culture-Hive-case-study-Connies-Colander-dementia.pdf

Libraries Connected (n.d.) *Universal Health Offer Infographic*, www.librariesconnected.org.uk/resource/universal-health-offer-infographic

Lin, Y., Chu, H., Yang, C. H., Chen, C. H., Chen, S. G., Chang, H. J. et al. (2011) Effectiveness of Group Music Intervention Against Agitated Behavior in Elderly Persons with Dementia, *International Journal of Geriatric Psychiatry*, **26** (7), 670–8.

Longden E., Davis, P., Billington, J., Lampropoulou, S., Farrington, G., Magee, F., Walsh, E. and Corcoran, R. (2015) Shared Reading: Assessing the Intrinsic Value of a Literature-based Health Intervention, *Medical Humanities*, **41** (2), 113–20.

Longden, E., Davis, P., Carroll, J. and Billington, J. (2016) *Read to Care: An Investigation into Quality of Life Benefits of Shared Reading Groups for People Living with Dementia*, The Reader, www.thereader.org.uk/read-care-investigation-quality-life-benefits-shared-reading-groups-people-living-dementia

Lopez, R. (2020) Prisoners in US Suffering Dementia May Hit 200,000 Within the Next Decade – Many Won't Even Know Why They are Behind Bars, *The Conversation*, 25 June, https://theconversation.com/prisoners-in-us-suffering-dementia-may-hit-200-000-within-the-next-decade-many-wont-even-know-why-they-are-behind-bars-138236

Low, L. F. and Purwaningrum, F. (2020) Negative Stereotypes, Fear and Social Distance: A Systematic Review of Depictions of Dementia in Popular Culture in the Context of Stigma, *BMC Geriatrics*, **20** (1), 477.

Manca, R., De Marco, M. and Venneri, A. (2020) The Impact of COVID-19 Infection and Enforced Prolonged Social Isolation on Neuropsychiatric Symptoms in Older Adults With and Without Dementia: A Review, *Frontiers in Psychiatry*, **11**, 585540.

MancLibraries Blog (2022) *PlayList for Life in Age Friendly Manchester Libraries*, 20 January, https://manclibraries.blog/2022/01/20/playlist-for-life-in-age-friendly-manchester-libraries

Martynova, T. A., Orlova, E. V. and Kitaeva, E. M. (2020) How to Overcome Complexities of Interdisciplinary Communication? Translation from One Disciplinary Language into Another for Interdisciplinary Course Design, *Universal Journal of Educational Research*, **8** (4), 1185–91.

Masterson-Algar, P., Allen, M. C., Hyde, M., Keating, N. and Windle, G. (2021) Exploring the Impact of COVID-19 on the Care and Quality of Life of People with Dementia and their Carers: A Scoping Review, *Dementia*, **21** (2), 648–76.

McLean, J. (2011) *An Evidence Review of the Impact of Participatory Arts on Older People*, Mental Health Foundation.

McMillan, A. and McNicol, S. (2019) The Playful Space of Workshops: On Imagination, Improvisation and Ignoring Instrumentalism, *Writing in Practice*, **5**, www.nawe.co.uk/DB/current-wip-edition-2/articles/the-playful-space-of-workshops-on-imagination-improvisation-and-ignoring-instrumentalism.html

McNicol, S. (2008) *Joint-use Libraries*, Chandos.

McNicol, S. and Dalton, P. (2021) *Reading is Caring – Evaluation Report*, Birmingham City University, www.scottishbooktrust.com/reading-and-stories/reading-is-caring/reading-is-caring-evaluation

McNicol, S. and Leamy, C. (2020) Co-creating a Graphic Illness Narrative with People with Dementia, *Journal of Applied Arts & Health*, **11** (3), 267–80.

Mitchell, W. (2018) *Somebody I Used to Know*, Bloomsbury.

Ministerio de Salud (2017) *Plan Nacional de Demencia [National Dementia Plan]*, Gobierno de Chile, www.minsal.cl/wp-content/uploads/2017/11/PLAN-DE-DEMENCIA.pdf

Molyneux, C., Hardy, T., Lin, Y. -Z. (C.), McKinnon, K. and Odell-Miller, H. (2020) Together in Sound: Music Therapy Groups for People with Dementia and Their Companions – Moving Online in Response to a Pandemic, *Approaches: An Interdisciplinary Journal of Music Therapy*.

Music For Dementia (n.d.) *Research and Evidence White Paper*, Music for Dementia, https://musicfordementia.org.uk/wp-content/uploads/2020/12/Music-for-Dementia-research-White-Paper.pdf

National Institute for Health and Care Excellence (NICE) (2018) *Dementia: Assessment, Management and Support for People Living with Dementia and their Carers* (NG97), NICE, www.nice.org.uk/guidance/ng97

Neuroscience Research Australia (NeuRA) (2019) Caring for Spirit: Aboriginal and Torres Strait Islander Online Dementia Education, https://caringforspirit.neura.edu.au

Nichols, E. and GBD 2019 Dementia Forecasting Collaborators (2019) Estimation of the Global Prevalence of Dementia in 2019 and Forecasted Prevalence in 2050: An Analysis for the Global Burden of Disease Study 2019, *The Lancet Public Health*, **7** (2), e105–e125.

O'Shea, E., Hopper, L., Marques, M., Gonçalves-Pereira, M., Woods, B., Jelley, H. et al. (2020) A Comparison of Self and Proxy Quality of Life Ratings for People with Dementia and their Carers: A European Prospective Cohort Study, *Aging & Mental Health*, **24** (1), 162–70.

Pani-Harreman, K., Bours, G., Zander, I., Kempen, G. and Van Duren, J. (2021) Definitions, Key Themes and Aspects of 'Ageing in Place': A Scoping Review. *Ageing and Society*, **41**, 2026–59.

Pictures to Share (n.d.) *How to Get Most from Our Books*, www.picturestoshare.co.uk/how-to-guide

Playlist for Life (2019) *Playlist for Life*, www.playlistforlife.org.uk

Postlethwaite, L. (2021) *Treasury of Arts Activities for Older People, Volume* 2, Baring Foundation.

Public Health Agency of Canada (2019) *A Dementia Strategy for Canada: Together We Aspire*, Government of Canada, www.canada.ca/en/public-health/services/publications/diseases-conditions/dementia-strategy.html

Ritchie, L., Tolson, D. and Danson, M. (2017) Dementia in the Workplace Case Study Research: Understanding the Experiences of Individuals, Colleagues and Managers, *Ageing and Society*, **38**, 2146–75.

Roche, M., Higgs, P., Aworinde, J. and Cooper, C. (2021) A Review of Qualitative Research of Perception and Experiences of Dementia Among Adults from Black, African, and Caribbean Background: What and Whom Are We Researching?, *Gerontologist*, **61** (5), e195–e208.

Rodrigues e Silva, A. M., Geldsetzer, F., Holdorff, B., Kielhorn, F. W., Balzer-Geldsetzer, M., Oertel, W. H., Hurtig, H. and Dodel, R. (2010) Who Was the Man who Discovered the 'Lewy bodies'?, *Movement Disorders*, **25** (12), 1765–73.

Ryan, N. S., Rossor, M. N. and Fox, N. C. (2015) Alzheimer's Disease in the 100 Years Since Alzheimer's Death, *Brain*, **138** (12), 3816–21.

Sagbakken, M., Ingebretsen, R. and Spilker, R. S. (2020) How to Adapt Caring Services to Migration-driven Diversity? A Qualitative Study Exploring Challenges and Possible Adjustments in the Care of People Living with Dementia, *PLoS ONE*, **15** (12), e0243803.

Sánchez, A., Millán-Calenti, J. C., Lorenzo-López, L. and Maseda, A. (2013) Multisensory Stimulation for People with Dementia: A Review of the Literature, *American Journal of Alzheimer's Disease and Other Dementias*, **28**, 7–14.

Savla, J., Roberto, K. A., Blieszner, R., McCann, B. R., Hoyt, E. and Knight, A. L. (2021) Dementia Caregiving During the 'Stay-at-Home' Phase of COVID-19 Pandemic, *The Journals of Gerontology Series B, Psychological Sciences and Social Sciences*, **76** (4), e241–e245.

Scottish Book Trust (2022), *Reading is Caring*, www.scottishbooktrust.com/reading-and-stories/reading-is-caring

Sefton Council (2022) *Sefton's Lost Voices*, www.sefton.gov.uk/schools-learning/libraries/local-archives-and-history-information-services/seftons-lost-voices

Shared Intelligence (2017) *Stand By Me: The Contribution of Public Libraries to the Well-being of Older People*, Arts Council England.

Shropshire Libraries (n.d.) *Oswestry Memory Loss Collection*, https://shropshire.gov.uk/media/18666/omlc-catalogue.pdf

Silko, L. M. (2012) *Storyteller*, Penguin.

Simonetti, A., Pais, C., Jones, M., Cipriani, M. C., Janiri, D., Monti, L. et al. (2020) Neuropsychiatric Symptoms in Elderly With Dementia During COVID-19 Pandemic: Definition, Treatment, and Future Directions, *Frontiers in Psychiatry*, **11**, 579842.

Social Care Institute for Excellence (SCIE) (2019) *Dementia Awareness E-learning Course*, www.scie.org.uk/e-learning/dementia

Social Care Institute for Excellence (SCIE) (2020a) *Dementia: At a Glance*, www.scie.org.uk/dementia/about

Social Care Institute for Excellence (SCIE) (2020b) *Creative Arts for People with Dementia*, www.scie.org.uk/dementia/living-with-dementia/keeping-active/creative-arts.asp

Social Care Institute for Excellence (SCIE) (2020c) *Reminiscence for People with Dementia*, www.scie.org.uk/dementia/living-with-dementia/keeping-active/reminiscence.asp

Social Care Institute for Excellence (SCIE) (2020d) *The Person Behind the Dementia*, www.scie.org.uk/dementia/after-diagnosis/communication/person.asp

South West Yorkshire Partnership NHS Foundation Trust (2022) *Cook and Eat Easy Read Books*, www.southwestyorkshire.nhs.uk/get-involved/eyup-charity/support-eyup/cook-and-eat-easy-read-books

Sporting Memories (n.d.) *About Our Clubs*, www.sportingmemoriesnetwork.com/Pages/FAQs/Category/our-clubs

Stockton Information Directory (n.d.) *Local History Group for People with Dementia – Stockton Reference Library*, www.stocktoninformationdirectory.org/kb5/stockton/directory/service.page?id=ra4mSy_G6xY&adultchannel=0#

Suárez-González, A., Livingston, G., Low, L. F., Cahill, S., Hennelly, N., Dawson, W. D. et al. (2020) *Impact and Mortality of COVID-19 on People Living with Dementia: Cross-country Report*, International Long-Term Care Policy Network.

Tales and Travel (n.d.) *Tales and Travel Memory Programs*, http://talesandtravelmemories.com

The National Archives (n.d.) *Connecting through Collections*, www.nationalarchives.gov.uk/education/outreach/projects/connecting-through-collections

The Reading Agency (2022) *Reading Well: Dementia*, https://reading-well.org.uk/books/books-on-prescription/dementia

The Reading Agency and Society of Chief Librarians (2013) *Reading Well Books on Prescription Scheme for People with Dementia and Their Families and Carers: Consultation Paper*, The Reading Agency.

Torack, R. (1983) The Early History of Senile Dementia. In Reisberg, B. (ed), *Alzheimer's Disease: The Standard Reference,* New York Free Press, 23–8.

Toronto Public Library (2020) *Pieces of History: 70 Digital Puzzle of Items in Our Special Collections,* https://torontopubliclibrary.typepad.com/local-history-genealogy/2020/05/pieces-of-history-35-digital-puzzles-of-items-in-our-special-collections.html

Touchstone (2022) *BME Dementia Service,* https://touchstonesupport.org.uk/community-services/bme-dementia-service

Tyler, A. (2020) *Health on the Shelf,* Scottish Library and Information Council (SLiC), https://scottishlibraries.org/media/3008/health-on-the-shelf.pdf

United Nations Department of Economic and Social Affairs (UN DESA) (2022) *Convention on the Rights of Persons with Disabilities (CRPD),* UN DESA, www.un.org/development/desa/disabilities/convention-on-the-rights-of-persons-with-disabilities.html

University of Bradford (2022) *Dementia Care Mapping,* www.bradford.ac.uk/dementia/training-consultancy/dcm

Vaitheswaran, S., Lakshminarayanan, M., Ramanujam, V., Sargunan, S. and Venkatesan, S. (2020) Experiences and Needs of Caregivers of Persons with Dementia in India during the COVID-19 Pandemic – A Qualitative Study, *American Journal of Geriatric Psychiatry,* **28** (11), 1185–94.

Vestavia Hills Library in the Forest (2022) *Cognitive Care Kits,* https://vestavialibrary.org/cognitive-care-kits

Walsall Healthcare NHS Trust (2019) *Distraction Therapy Collection,* www.walsallhealthcare.nhs.uk/professionals/library/i-would-like/loan-equipment/distraction-therapy-collection

Walworth, R. M. (2018) Adapting the Books on Prescription Model for People Living with Dementia and their Carers. In McNicol, S. and Brewster, L. (eds), *Bibliotherapy,* Facet Publishing, 163–70.

Williams, G. and Farmer, J. (2016) Old, Grey and Locked Away: CST Group Work in Prison, *Journal of Dementia Care,* **24** (1), 12–14.

Wilkinson, H. (2002) *The Perspectives of People with Dementia: Research Methods and Motivations,* Jessica Kingsley Publishers.

Wisconsin Alzheimer's Institute (2017) *Dementia Friendly Libraries in Wisconsin: A Best Practice Guide,* Wisconsin Alzheimer's Institute, University of Wisconsin, https://dfmassachusetts.org/wp-content/uploads/sites/6/2019/06/Dementia-Friendly-Libraries-in-Wisconsin-A-Best-Practice-Guide.pdf

Woods, B., Aguirre, E., Spector, A. E. and Orrell, M. (2012) Cognitive Stimulation to Improve Cognitive Functioning in People with Dementia, *Cochrane Database of Systematic Reviews,* **2** (2), CD005562.

Woods, B., O'Philbin, L., Farrell, E. M., Spector, A. E. and Orrell, M. (2018) Reminiscence Therapy for Dementia, *Cochrane Database of Systematic Reviews*, **3** (3), CD001120.

World Health Organisation (WHO) (2019) *Risk Reduction of Cognitive Decline and Dementia: WHO Guidelines*, World Health Organization.

World Health Organization (WHO) (2021) Dementia: Key Facts, www.who.int/news-room/fact-sheets/detail/dementia

Zeilig, H., Killick, J. and Fox, C. (2014) The Participative Arts for People Living with a Dementia: A Critical Review, *International Journal of Ageing and Later Life*, **9** (1), 7–34.

Annotated Bibliography

This annotated bibliography provides links to resources that may be useful for libraries wishing to explore ways to make their provision more dementia friendly. It focuses on practical guidelines and tools. If you want to explore research, policy documents, etc., please take a look at the literature included in the References section.

National dementia and Alzheimer's societies

Dementia or Alzheimer's societies in different parts of the world provide information and support specific to their national or regional context, but they are also worth exploring if you are from another country as much of the information about dementia and supporting people to live well with the condition will be applicable regardless of location. It is also worth noting that most organisations for Alzheimer's will provide information about other types of dementia too. The following list is far from exhaustive, but these are some of the organisations I've gathered information from whilst researching this book.

Alzheimer Society of Canada: https://alzheimer.ca/en
Alzheimer's Association, US: www.alz.org
Alzheimer's Disease International: www.alzint.org
Alzheimer's New Zealand: https://alzheimers.org.nz
Alzheimer's Scotland: www.alzscot.org
Alzheimer Society of Ireland: https://alzheimer.ie
Alzheimer's Society UK: www.alzheimers.org.uk
Dementia Australia: www.dementia.org.au
Dementia UK: www.dementiauk.org

Understanding dementia

These resources may be helpful to better understand various aspects of dementia.

A Walk Through Dementia

www.awalkthroughdementia.org
An app developed by Alzheimer's Research UK and guided by people living with different forms of dementia to help those without dementia to understand what everyday life can be like for people with the condition. It features three everyday situations: a supermarket, travelling and home. Each demonstrates challenges people with dementia may face.

Alzheimer's Research UK

www.alzheimersresearchuk.org
Alzheimer's Research UK is the UK's leading dementia research charity, dedicated to research into causes, diagnosis, prevention, treatment and cure. Their website has information about dementia, in particular the medical aspects of the condition, in understandable language for a variety of audiences.

Patient.info

https://patient.info/brain-nerves/memory-loss-and-dementia
An online health information directory of evidence-based clinical information for medical staff and their patients. There is a section about dementia with articles on a range of topics.

Social Care Institute for Excellence (SCIE) resource hub

www.scie.org.uk/dementia
A resource hub for anyone supporting people with dementia. Many of the resources are for people working in social care but may also be relevant for staff in other organisations, such as libraries.

Young Dementia Network

www.youngdementianetwork.org
A UK-based community of people living with young-onset dementia, their family and friends, as well as professionals in health and social care and the voluntary sector.

Creating a Dementia-friendly Workplace: A Practical Guide for Employers

Alzheimer's Society (2015)

www.alzheimers.org.uk/sites/default/files/migrate/downloads/creating_a_dementia-friendly_workplace.pdf

This guide for employers is designed to help them provide support for staff members with dementia. It may also be a useful resource for people living with, or affected by, dementia in the workplace. Whilst written for a UK context, the guide includes practical tips that are relevant more broadly.

Dementia-friendly design

Resources providing guidance on the design of dementia-friendly buildings and spaces.

Dementia Friendly Design Tool

Dementia Services Development Centre/Kirklees Council (2021)

www.kirklees.gov.uk/beta/health-and-well-being/pdf/kirklees-dementia-design-guide.pdf

This Dementia-Friendly Design Tool, introduced into Kirklees in the UK, is a collection of guidance that supports dementia-friendly design, layout and furnishing of buildings and spaces. It includes a section specific to libraries that comprises general guidance and a checklist to identify specific elements that can contribute to dementia-friendly design.

Tips for Dementia-friendly Spaces

Dementia-Friendly Canada

https://alzheimer.ca/sites/default/files/documents/DFC-Spaces%20TipSheet_Final.pdf

A simple, well laid out checklist to assess workplace environments and develop action plans for making spaces more dementia friendly.

Is this INSIDE Public Space Dementia-inclusive? A Checklist for Use by Dementia Groups

Innovations in Dementia CIC, ECRED (University of Edinburgh) and Dementia Centre HammondCare (2017)

www.dementiavoices.org.uk/wp-content/uploads/2017/09/Inside-checklist.pdf

A checklist designed for dementia groups to use to assess the dementia friendliness of a public building. This is detailed and accessible, but if you are thinking of using this checklist, I would recommend changing the 'Action needed' column to a more straightforward 'Yes/No' and minor editing to ensure all statements are phrased positively (for example, Question 5 includes both 'loud music' (negative) and 'quiet times advertised' (positive) in the same list).

Reminiscence resources

There are a number of websites that provide images, audio and video resources that may be useful for reminiscence (or for imaginative activities such as storytelling) with people with dementia. I have focused on UK resources as access may be limited by country, but there will be similar resources available in most regions.

BBC Reminiscence Archive (RemArc)

https://remarc.bbcrewind.co.uk

This archive provides access to a selection of content from the BBC Archives designed to support reminiscence. You can access resources via theme (such as sport, events, etc.) or decade (1930s, 1940s, etc.) and choose image, audio or video content. The layout is very simple, making it potentially accessible for people with early-stage dementia to interact with the site themselves. Most clips are short, many under a minute in length, so likely to maintain engagement. Items can be 'favourited' to return to later.

BBC Music Memories

https://musicmemories.bbcrewind.co.uk/home

A simple website to allow you to build a playlist, with selections for decades, countries, languages and composers. There are also theme tunes and a social music section that includes pub songs, football songs and religious music. You can hear extracts on the site and playlists can be exported to Spotify to listen in full. There is also a memory radio section with clips from BBC Radio by decade and region of the UK.

BFI Player

https://player.bfi.org.uk/free

BFI Player is a video on demand service from the British Film Institute, streaming a large number of archive films. Many are available for free, although access is limited to the UK. Films available range in length from a couple of minutes to full length films and include newsreels, adverts, films produced by cultural institutions and amateur filmmakers.

National Library of Wales' 'Living Memory' scheme
www.library.wales/livingmemory
The aim of the Living Memory scheme is to utilise The National Library of Wales' graphic and audio-visual collections to facilitate reminiscence with older people and those living with dementia. Packs of photographs and films have been compiled for use by community and voluntary groups, day centres, care homes and health establishments throughout Wales. These resources are offered free of charge to public libraries and those working in elderly care and mental health care.

House of Memories, Liverpool Museums
www.liverpoolmuseums.org.uk/house-of-memories/my-house-of-memories-app
House of Memories started with the collections of the Museum of Liverpool in the UK but has since worked with museums across the UK and internationally. The House of Memories app is designed to be easy to use for people with dementia and their carers. It has pictures of objects from across the decades, together with sound, music and descriptions. Objects are organised by theme, such as school, work, leisure and maritime, and there are collections specific to the US and Singapore, as well as the UK. Users can save favourite objects to a digital memory tree, digital memory box or timeline. The app also has a 'My Memories' feature, which enables users to upload their own photos and add their own notes.

Other activities
National Activity Providers Association (NAPA)
https://napa-activities.co.uk/services/resources/free-resources
NAPA is a membership organisation for providers of care and support services for adults in the UK. It offers a variety of resources and training opportunities for members, but also has some useful free resources with ideas for activities.

The Baring Foundation
Treasury of arts activities for older people (Vols 1 & 2), compiled by Liz Postlethwaite
https://baringfoundation.org.uk/resource/treasury-of-arts-activities-for-older-people
https://baringfoundation.org.uk/resource/treasury-of-arts-activities-for-older-people-volume-2
These are published collections of arts activities designed for older people. Many of the activities are dementia friendly and there are both one-to-one and group activities.

Dementia Friendly Screenings
www.cinemauk.org.uk/wp-content/uploads/2017/10/Dementia-Friendly-Screenings_Guide_for_cinemas.pdf
Guidance for cinemas offering dementia-friendly screenings, but also helpful for libraries and other venues offering film screenings.

Language and dementia
There are a number of guidelines on the use of language in relation to dementia and people living with the condition. Whilst the overall messages are broadly consistent, there are differences in details of the guidance depending on the local context in different countries. The following are some examples.

Dementia Language Guidelines, Dementia Australia
www.dementia.org.au/sites/default/files/resources/dementia-language-guidelines.pdf

Person-centred Language Guidelines, Alzheimer's Society of Canada
https://alzheimer.ca/sites/default/files/documents/Person-centred-language-guidelines_Alzheimer-Society.pdf

Positive Language: An Alzheimer's Society Guide to Talking About Dementia, Alzheimer's Society UK
www.alzheimers.org.uk/sites/default/files/2018-09/Positive%20language%20guide_0.pdf

Dementia Words Matter: Guidelines on Language About Dementia, DEEP (The Dementia Engagement and Empowerment Project, UK)
http://dementiavoices.org.uk/wp-content/uploads/2013/11/DEEP-Guide-Writing-dementia-friendly-information.pdf

Communications guidelines
Designing for Dementia, AbilityNet, UK
https://abilitynet.org.uk/factsheets/designing-dementia

Age-positive Image Library, Centre for Ageing Better
https://ageingbetter.resourcespace.com/pages/home.php

Writing Dementia-friendly Information, DEEP (The Dementia Engagement and Empowerment Project, UK)
DEEP-Guide-Writing-dementia-friendly-information.pdf

Creating Websites for People with Dementia, DEEP (The Dementia Engagement and Empowerment Project, UK)
http://dementiavoices.org.uk/wp-content/uploads/2013/11/DEEP-Guide-Creating-websites.pdf

Evaluation and research methods
Methods@Manchester
www.methods.manchester.ac.uk/themes
Videos, presentations and other resources on a range of research methods.

Introduction to Visual Research Methods
https://drive.google.com/file/d/1gKf9EajbNsU-WjMMJb68dEMuwUfj-wnf/view

Index

age-friendly communities 27
ageing in place 150
   community circles 150
   local area co-ordination 150
Alzheimer's disease xix–xxi, 1, 3–4, 64, 144
   atypical Alzheimer's 4, 8
   causes xx, 3
   history xix–xx
   prevalence 3, xx–xxi, 144
   symptoms 3–4
archives 98–9
   digital jigsaws 105–6
   The National Archives 103–4
   Stockton Local History Archive 89–90, 99
arts-based activities 18–19, 92–9, 103–5, 115, 118
   co-authorship 97
   creative writing 96–7
   film screenings 94–5
   mark making 96–7
   music 92–4, 97, 102–3
   online 102–5
   poetry 59, 66, 70, 72, 97
   singing 60, 82, 93–4, 105
   storytelling 95–6
   theatre 94–5

bibliotherapy 58, 69–79, 118
   one-to-one 75–8
   reading groups 69–75
   The Reader 70
   Reading is Caring 75–8, 108–9, 120
   research 58
   shared reading 70–1, 75–7
   Words in Mind 71–4, 118
Booktrust 63
built environment *see* library design

calm rooms 54
care homes xx, 51, 107, 111–12, 115–20
   arts activities 96–7
   Belong Crewe xiv, 96, 149
   communications 117–19
   Halton Libraries' reminiscence box service 116–18
   language 119–20
   partnerships 115–20
   reading groups 72–4, 118
   reminiscence 99, 116–18
   Sefton's Lost Voices 98–9, 118–19
   staff training 37, 118
   Words in Mind 72–4, 118
carers xx, xxii, 32, 34–5, 145, 148
   impact of COVID-19 xv, 151
   library-based activities 86, 95, 153
   online activities 69, 107–9
   reading groups 69
   research participation 130, 132, 135
   terminology xxviii, 124–5
   training 37, 76, 108–9
cognitive care kits 91
   Akron-Summit County Public Library 91
   Vestavia Hills Library in the Forest 91
Cognitive Stimulation Therapy 82–3
   Norwich Prison Library 82–3
collection development 69, 84, 97–9
   involving people with dementia 97–9

Sefton's Lost Voices 98–9
Stockton-on-Tees reminiscence collection 99
comics 14, 64–5, 97
  co-authorship 14, 97
  reactions to 64–5
  Tangles 64–5
communication 12–13, 28–31, 121–8
  7Cs of communication 125–6
  design 125–7
  images 126
  language 87, 122–5
  media 127
  online 103
  tips 29–30
  translation 127
  verbal 28–31
  written 125–7
Connie's Colander 95
COVID-19 xv, 151
  care homes 51, 116–7, 151
  impacts 93, 101, 135
    on carers xv; on people with dementia xv, 151
  isolation xv
  technology use 69, 101–5, 108–9
CST *see* Cognitive Stimulation Therapy
customer service 28–32
  communication 29–31
  training 36–9, 113–14

delusions 12
dementia xix–xxxvii, 1–19
  café *see* memory café
  care models 150
  history xix–xx
  fictional representation xxiii–xxiv, 64
  impact on library use 14–15
  library staff with 33–4
  living well with xx, xxiv–xxv, 21
  media representation 123, 127
  positive 25–6
  prevalence xx–xxi, 143–5
  social interaction 86–7
  stages of 9–10
  stigma xxi–xxii, 122–3, 148
  symptoms 1–2, 9–14

Dementia Australia staff recommend sticker 62–3
dementia-friendly communities 24–8, 38
  recognition 26
Dementia Friendly Toolkit for Libraries 27–8
Dementia Services Development Centre 42, 47
  Dementia-Friendly Design Tool 49–50
distraction therapy 84
  Walsall NHS Trust Library 84
doll therapy 85–6
  Bedford Free Public Library 86
Dovetale Press 66

ethnicity 144–8
  immigrant communities 145–6
  indigenous communities 124, 146–8
evaluation 129–42
  emotional touchpoints 137
  focus groups 138–9
  interviews 134–8
    online 135–6; types of 134–5; walking 137–8
  surveys 132–3
  talking mats 140
  visual methods 139–40

focus groups 138–9
frontotemporal dementia 7–8
  symptoms 7–8
  types 7

hallucinations 2, 4, 10
Healthybooks 64

interviewing 134–8

Kitwood, Tom xiv, xxiv, 15–17
  model of psychological needs 16, 74, 77, 83, 131

language 119–20, 122–5, 127, 146–7
  carer 124–5
  person with dementia 122–4
Lewy body dementia xx, 6–7
  causes 6
  dementia with Lewy bodies 6

Parkinson's disease dementia 6
prevalence 6
symptoms 7
LGBT+ communities 148–9
Silver Pride 149, 154
library design 41–55
  access 43
  Almondbury Library 50
  Belper Library 51
  colour 42, 46
  Deichman Oppsal Library 51–2
  dementia-friendly 42–52
  Dementia-Friendly Design Tool 49–50
  furnishing 46
  Great Sankey Neighbourhood Hub 47–8
  Kirklees Libraries 49–50
  lighting 43, 46, 85
  multi-function facility 43, 47–8, 114–15
  Sandal Library 50–1
  signage 42–4, 55
  Stockton Heath library 48–9
  Warrington (Livewire) Libraries 47–9
library staff 28–9, 32–9, 41, 45, 48–9, 54–5
  as carers 34–5
  training for 36–9, 113–14
  with dementia 33–4
life story work 76, 120
  book boxes 76, 78, 120
living well with dementia xx, xxiv–xxv, 21
local studies *see* archives
Local Dementia Action Alliance 112–13

magic table 106–7, 115–16
  Guernsey Libraries 106–7, 115–16
MCI *see* mild cognitive impairment
memory café 53–4, 87–8
  languages 87, 146
  Let's Talk dementia social group 87–8
memory boxes 76, 117, 120
mild cognitive impairment 9
misidentification 12
misperceptions 11
mixed dementia 8
Montessori book clubs 74–5

outreach activities 103–5, 115–19

Guernsey Libraries 106–7, 115–16
Halton Libraries' reminiscence box service 116–18
online 103–5
Sefton's Lost Voices 98–9, 118–19

Parkinson's disease xx, 6
partnerships 111–20
  care homes 115–20
  challenges 114–20
  co-location of services 47–8, 114–15
  Halton Libraries' reminiscence box service 116–18
  Local Dementia Action Alliances 112–13
  media 127
  North Shore Library Memory Connection Center 113–14
  Safe Places 113
  Sefton's Lost Voices 118–19
person-centred care 15–19
  creative arts practice 18–19
  guidelines and standards 18
  personal enhancers 17–18
personhood 15–16
Pictures to Share 65–8
Playlist for Life 93
  AK Bell library 93
portals 63
  East Cheshire NHS Trust Library and Knowledge Service 63
prison libraries 82–3
  Norwich Prison Library 82–3

quiet hour 84–5
  Kingsfold Public Library 85
  Manchester Libraries 85
  South Taranaki Libraries 85

reading 57–79
  children and young people 63–4
  easy readers 65–6
  external texts 59–60
  groups 69–75
  imagination 58–9, 78, 153
  internal texts 59–60
  Montessori book clubs 74–5
  picture books 65–6

The Reader 70–1
Reading is Caring 75–8, 108–9, 120
recommendation schemes 61–3
shared 70–1, 75–7
step-by-step books 66–7
Tales and Travel Memories 71
texts 57, 59–60, 78
Words in Mind 59, 71–4, 118, 154
Reading is Caring 75–8, 108–9
  online workshops 120
Reading Well Books on Prescription for Dementia 61–2
reminiscence 88–91, 99
  Halton Libraries' reminiscence box service 116–18
  memory boxes 76, 117, 120
  Shropshire Libraries' shared memory bags 67–8
  Sporting Memories Clubs 90–1
  Stockton Local History Group 89–90, 123–4
research 129–42
  ethics 140–1
  into dementia xv, xxi–xxii, 57–8, 82, 88, 102–3, 145, 148
  with carers 32, 34–5, 132, 135
  with people with dementia 129–42
restlessness 13
rights-based approach 23–4

Scottish Book Trust 75, 108
sensory hour *see* quiet hour
sensory spaces 53–4
  immersive experience room 53–4
service development *see* evaluation
shared reading 70–1, 75–7
  The Reader 70–1
  Reading is Caring 75–7
singing 60, 82, 93–4, 105
  Norfolk Library and Information Service 105
  online 102, 105
  Shropshire Libraries 93–4
Snoezelen therapy 53
social activities 86–91
  cognitive care kits 91
  Let's Talk Dementia Social Group 87–8

memory cafes 87–8
reminiscence 88–91
Sporting Memories Clubs 90–1
Stockton Local History Group 89–90, 123–4
social model of disability 22–3
Sporting Memories Clubs 90–1
surveys 132–3

Tales and Travel Memories 71
technology 89–90, 101–10, 115–16, 151
  arts workshops 103–4
  carers 69, 107–9
  COVID-19 69, 101–3, 153
  digital jigsaws 105–6
  guidance 102–3
  magic table 106–7, 115–16
  Makewrite app 97
  music therapy 102
  online dementia action week 108
  singing groups 102, 105
  Toronto Public Library 106
  video conferencing 102–5, 108–9
  virtual reality 151
time-shifting 11
Tovertafel *see* magic table
training 34, 36–9, 108–9, 113–14 118
  care home staff 108–9, 118
  Dementia-Friendly Canada 38–9
  Dementia Friends 36–7
  online 37–9, 108–9
  Social Care Institute of Excellence 37
  Wisconsin Libraries 37, 113–14

vascular dementia 5–6
  causes 5
  prevalence 5
  symptoms 5–6
  types 5
visual research 139–40
volunteers 34–5, 63, 68, 72–3, 93, 98

Where the Arts Belong 96
Words in Mind 59, 71–4, 118, 154

young-onset dementia 8–9, 27
  prevalence 8